This book is an invitation to make sure that we are in charge of technology rather than technology being in charge of us. It is a wonderful gift for anyone who wants to take a step back and explore the question: How do I want to live my life? In meeting that question with curiosity, we examine our relationship with nature, technology, body, mind, and spirit in the context of community.

— René Molenkamp, PhD
Co-founder and Executive Director of Group Relations International

In their lively and inspiring new book, *Experience Nature Unplugged*, Sonya Mohamed and Sebastian Slovin have shown us the way back to the pleasures and necessity of being active bodies connected to nature. They offer convincing data for making a conscious shift from overentanglement with the virtual world to a more organic and mindful existence in the natural world—which is, by the way, our true home.

— Emma Mellon, PhD
Licensed Psychologist and Author

Experience Nature Unplugged addresses the biggest problem we face today—our overreliance on devices—by offering strategies to shift our mindset and re-create our relationship with technology. It's an integrated approach that incorporates leadership, wellness, and the healing power of the outdoors. This book is for all of us, parents, teachers, leaders ... anyone who knows a more meaningful life awaits us when we put down our devices.

— Lorri Sulpizio, PhD
Director of Conscious Leadership Academy

A refreshing blend of big-picture inspiration and very practical steps for developing healthier relationships to social media, nature, and one's deeper self. If taken to heart, the guidance offered will be life changing. It's a gift to yourself to read it.

— Theresa (Terri) Monroe, RSCJ, EdD
Associate Professor of Leadership Studies

Experience Nature Unplugged is a must-read! This is the perfect prescription for health and wellness in the digital age.

— Mark Kalina, MD

I was initially struck by the balance between the compelling personal stories of the two authors, the depth of their vision and the detailed, practical, holistic "operations manual" they have created. A significant amount of personal experience and research is condensed, digested, and integrated in a way that illuminates the challenges of 21st-century life and the promise of a life in balance.

— Jack Lampl
Organizational Consultant, Past President of the A. K. Rice Institute

Sebastian and Sonya provide a step-by-step plan for finding a healthy and balanced relationship with technology and all the benefits attained through connecting with nature. I recommend it for anyone that wants to live the most intentional, impactful, and aware life possible. You should read this book and then go Experience Nature Unplugged!

— Derek Abbey, PhD
President and CEO of Project Recover

Experience Nature Unplugged inspires and offers insight on how to balance our digital world with our natural world. Sebastian and Sonya's life experiences and creativity anchor a deep and relevant list of resources that steer the reader toward the recognition that nature is our heart and soul, and that without it, our health and outlook become disengaged, stressed, and disconnected. The activities and reflections make the book experience come to life and offer us a mirror into ourselves and our habits, all while empowering us to make meaningful changes to our daily routines.

— Diana Richardson
Faculty Emeritus, Geography, San Diego State University

Finally, a calm, sensible, and effective approach to our hyperconnected, anxious, and overstimulated lifestyle. The best part is that they give us the tools to create more balance in our lives without using fear or guilt as motivators.

— Monica Stapleton, LMFT
Founder of Disconnect Collective

EXPERIENCE
NATURE UNPLUGGED

A GUIDE TO WELLNESS
IN THE DIGITAL AGE

SEBASTIAN SLOVIN
&
SONYA MOHAMED

Nature Unplugged – Encinitas, California – 2021

sebastian@natureunplugged.com, www.natureunplugged.com

Printed and bound in the United States of America
ISBN: 978-1-7363938-0-2
Library of Congress Control Number: 2021902149

Design & layout by Sonya Mohamed
Cover design by Isaac Mitchell
Cover photo by Annie Spratt

To Patti Fox,
With love and gratitude.

Your wild and courageous spirit lives on.

"What would our lives be like if our days and nights were as immersed in nature as they are in technology?"
—Richard Louv

PREFACE

What's the most valuable nonrenewable resource we have?

Time.

Time is such an interesting thing. It's our only truly nonrenewable resource, yet many of us live our day-to-day lives as if we have infinite amounts of time. It's often not until we're facing our own mortality from an accident, a challenging health condition, old age, or the death of someone close to us that we really get in touch with how valuable and limited our time here is. It's so easy to take it for granted.

Knowing that we're not guaranteed any certain amount of this precious resource, what do we want to do with the time we have?

Here at Nature Unplugged, this is often how we start the conversation about wellness in today's digital age. The challenging thing about time (especially in our high-tech world) is that if we're not proactive and intentional about how we use it, something else will fill that space, and our time gets used up either way. Every second we're making a choice about what we're doing, consciously or unconsciously, whether it's action or inaction. The way it's playing out for millions of people around the world is that their time is unintentionally taken up by scrolling through social media feeds, passively surfing the web, checking email, and being distracted by likes, dings, and all sorts of digital notifications.

Take a look around the next time you're in a restaurant or grocery store, or any public space, for that matter. People are glued to their screens and are often disengaged from themselves, other humans, and the world around them. Is that intentional behavior? The answer, most of the time, is no way! People aren't consciously thinking, *You know, it's been 30 seconds since I last checked Instagram. I'd better get back on there and see what's new. I hope I didn't miss anything important.* Our precious time is being swept away by unconscious habits and a lack of intentionality.

The issue of mindlessly scrolling our lives away isn't as straightforward as it may seem. It's complex and can be difficult to navigate. That's why so many of us get sucked into screen vortexes. The people creating the technology design it specifically to capture our time and attention and keep it for as long as possible. Knowing this, it's up to us to determine if that tech is helpful and serving our needs, or harmful and a distraction. Rather than harping on all the problems, this book focuses on the solutions. It can help you create a healthy relationship with technology and nature so that you can start spending your time doing the things that matter most to you. This book will give you and your community the tools to live with more intention and awareness. It's a how-to guide for wellness in the digital age.

CONTENTS

Part Five. Recharge: How to Harness the Power of Play
and Creativity

Experience Nature Unplugged

ℕ

You cannot teach a man anything,
you can only help him find it within himself.
—Galileo

Have you ever seen the Disney movie *Wall-E*? If not, we highly recommend it. Also, spoiler alert. Well, we'll try not to give too much away. The Pixar movie is about a distant future in which humans have used up all the resources on Earth. There are no plants or animals left, and Earth is a wasteland filled with the trash and remnants of the humans who once lived there. The main character in the movie is a little trash-collecting robot named Wall-E. For our purposes, the character Wall-E isn't too important. Our focus is on the remaining humans. They live on a giant spaceship that is searching the galaxies for a new planet to inhabit.

The way these future humans are portrayed would be hilarious if it wasn't so potentially realistic. They are soft and round and cruise around the spaceship on little personalized go-kart-like vehicles. The motorized carts have giant screens built in to provide constant entertainment. The humans also have access to any food and drink they want by the push of a button. These future people have been completely taken over by devices and technology—and they are almost entirely dependent on them. In fact, they can hardly walk or move around without the assistance of their vehicles. In essence, they are a depiction of what would probably happen if technology and convenience were to continue with no regard for things like human connection, nature, movement, and play (and many of the other things we will explore in this book).

While there's a big difference between our current state as a species and that of the people in *Wall-E*, that gap appears to be narrowing. The movie is a great reminder and motivation for us at Nature Unplugged. It is at the core of why we do what we do. Our aim is that *Wall-E* remains a fictional story and that we humans take a different path.

Our Relationship with Nature and Technology

Fortunately for us, we haven't quite reached the grim future of the people in *Wall-E* (yet) and we still have incredible natural resources here to enjoy. From the intricate design and detail of a tiny flower to the immense space in the open sky, there's so much beauty and wonder all around us. We live in an amazing world, yet many of us are paying more attention to our technology (devices, phones, and screens) than anything else. The natural world is in many ways the opposite of the digital world. If screens, wires, devices and outlets are on one end of the spectrum, then trees, clouds, and vast mountain ranges are on the other. And, as we will explore further, many of the negative outcomes from being overly connected to technology are remedied by time spent experiencing nature, unplugged.

To start, we must acknowledge that connection with nature is necessary for our survival and well-being as a species. Nature isn't something that is just nice to have or pretty to look at (although it is also that). It's our home and our habitat. It's an environment our species and DNA has known a great deal longer (historically speaking) than the digital world we live in today. Consider a brief timeline of our species. Anatomically modern humans have been roaming around Earth for about 200,000 years, and our earlier ancestors are estimated to have been around between five and seven million years ago. Civilization as we've come to know it only began around 6,000 years ago, and industrialization started in the 1800s. The digital revolution, which we're focusing on in this book, only began in the 1980s. This zoomed-out perspective of our history highlights that the digital age is a tiny blip on the timeline when compared to our species' total time on earth.

For the first time in history, people are spending more of their time inside, rarely and reluctantly venturing outdoors and into nature. We've become a community of indoor creatures who value comfort and convenience above most else. And we're suffering because of it, mentally, emotionally, and physically.

Why is this happening and what can we do about it?
What does a healthy relationship with technology look like?
What does a healthy relationship with nature look like?

These questions are at the core of the work we do at Nature Unplugged and are central to this book. Our mission is to inspire wellness in the digital age. In this book we'll explore the "why" behind society's obsessive dependence on smart devices and tech. We'll spend the rest of our time focusing on the solutions—on what we can do about it. But before we take another step on this journey together, we want to make it very clear that we are NOT anti-technology. In fact, we love technology! We (Sebastian and Sonya) live in the modern, high-tech world with all the wonderful conveniences that go with it. We don't live off the grid. We're not in a yurt in the middle of a forest. As we write this, we are enjoying and benefiting from technological advancements like electricity, lights, computers, smartphones and Wi-Fi.

That being said, when we step back and look at our lives (and the world around us), it seems like we've lost our way a bit. More specifically, we've lost our balance—the balance between enjoying and experiencing the conveniences of modern technology *and* enjoying and experiencing nature. As a society we've become more connected to our smart devices and less connected to ourselves, each other, and the world around us.

It's easy to wave a hand at that dismissively, and many have. But even if you think this problem, our overconnection to technology and disconnection from nature, seems minor, the effects and impact on our mental and physical health are enormous and concerning. This is not just our opinion, and we're not trying to be alarmist. There is an incredible amount of research to support the importance and necessity of time in nature for well-being. And while the research examining the impact of technology and screen time on humans is still relatively new, it's certainly gaining momentum, and the findings are worth paying attention to.

The Problem

To be clear, the problem is not technology. The challenge we're addressing is that we've become overly connected to technology and disconnected from ourselves, each other, and the natural world. This imbalance impacts our physical and mental health in myriad ways. To name a few, we're seeing higher instances of sedentary lifestyles, hypertension, obesity, and a decrease in strength on the physical health side. On the mental health side, we're seeing an increase in attention disorders, isolation, anxiety, depression, and suicide.

Here are a handful of statistics that help illustrate the problem:

- Tweens (9–12 years old) use 4.5 hours and teens use 7 hours of technology a day—not including time spent on school or homework.[1]
- People in the U.S. spend 90% of their time indoors.[2]
- 50% of teenagers "feel addicted" to their mobile device and 72% say they feel the need to immediately respond to texts and social networking messages.[3]
- Approximately 80% of adult smartphone users have their phones with them for 22 hours a day and check their phone within 15 minutes of waking up.[4]
- Childhood obesity increased from 7% in 1980 to 18% in 2015. Today, approximately 40% of adults in the U.S. are considered obese.[5]
- Teens and young adults who use social media intensely are as much as 66% more likely to report being depressed than casual users.[6]
- Preschool kids are the fastest-growing market for antidepressants.[7]

Research on the impact of increased technology use and screen time on our mental and physical well-being is piling up, with plenty of new literature written on this in recent years. There's a lot of information out there, but the aim of this book is *not* to focus solely on the problem or to give you an exhaustive list of why technology is bad (because again, it's not all bad). Instead, our goal is to help give you enough information to create a clear picture of what we're dealing with. What we're saying, in a nutshell, is that this isn't a literature review of all the research on the impact of technology use and benefits of nature. Once you know the basics of the problem, you'll have what you need to find meaningful solutions and a pathway forward—without getting sucked into a vortex of research. The majority of this book is dedicated to exploring ways to live well with technology and sharing practices, tips, and tools for bringing the balance back.

Why Read This Book

At Nature Unplugged we are all about wellness in the digital age. Since 2012, we've worked with thousands of clients—families, working professionals, educators, and students—through workshops, presentations, coaching, and retreats, helping them create healthy relationships with technology and reconnect to nature, themselves, and others. The purpose of this book is no different. These pages hold the same ideas, research, methods, and tools that have worked for our clients, and they are now available to you.

Breaking free from the clutches of technology overuse isn't just a nice idea. It's something that is absolutely achievable. We've experienced it ourselves, and we've seen it happen with the clients we work with every day. When we take back control of the devices in our lives, things start to shift and new possibilities open up. It's sort of like getting over a cold, where you didn't realize how bad you'd been feeling until you were all better. Or, not realizing how terrible your eyesight was before you got glasses and could see clearly. When we are able to rise above digital distractions and noise, we start to engage with life in a whole new way.

We have seen this transformation happen with our clients over and over again. Teenagers go from being sleep deprived, unfocused, and nearly flunking out of school because of social media and video game overuse to being engaged and driven to graduate. We've seen families go from being divided and at war over technology and screen time to being connected and on the same page. These changes didn't come from some miracle or incredible force of will but from making small changes, holding boundaries with tech, and creating space for the things that really bring them joy. When we free ourselves from tech overuse and the attention economy, all of a sudden there's more time in the day, deeper relationships with family and friends, and a renewed vigor and interest in life.

Why We Started Nature Unplugged

Before we move on, we want to take a moment to tell you who we are and why we do this work. We, Sebastian and Sonya, have had markedly different experiences and passions that have brought us to the point of writing this book together. Sebastian's background, both educational and professional, has been rooted in health, wellness, and nature. He holds a Bachelor of Arts in Environmental Policy from San Diego State University and a Master of Arts in Leadership Studies from the University of San Diego. He is also the author of *The Adventures of Enu*[8] and *Ashes in the Ocean*.[9] Sonya worked in higher education for more than 12 years, including for the University of North Carolina–Wilmington, Duke University, the University of California–Los Angeles, and most recently, the University of San Diego. She received a Master of Education in Student Affairs from the University of California–Los Angeles and a Master of Arts in Leadership Studies from the University of San Diego.

Sebastian is a San Diego native, while Sonya grew up in the Northeast. They've both enjoyed living across the U.S. and abroad but have recently made their home in the coastal town of Encinitas, California. They are partners in business and in life (aka married). That's who we are on the surface, but the energy and inspiration for the work we do comes from a much deeper place.

At a young age, Sebastian lost his father to suicide. This experience challenged him and changed him in many ways. One thing that came out of his loss was a renewed and deeper connection with nature, which lives on in his work today. Sonya spent much of her youth on track to becoming a soccer superstar. Her days were filled with practice, games, tournaments, and travel. Significant knee injuries before entering college and losing her father during her sophomore year changed her path, and she found a renewed sense of play and creative inspiration. It has been our backgrounds, as well as our research, that have shaped the work we do at Nature Unplugged.

Sebastian's Story

I was fortunate to grow up in La Jolla, a beautiful coastal town in Southern California. I had a pretty ideal upbringing, if I do say so myself. I spent a lot of time as a little tyke exploring the beach and the

6

sand and getting tumbled around in the shore break with my mom and dad and little sister. Many of my early memories were in and around the ocean with my dad. He was an incredible swimmer. He had grown up in South Africa and was one of the best butterfly swimmers in the world during his prime.

Some of my fondest memories of my dad are of swimming with him at the La Jolla Cove. I would hold onto his back as he'd swim out to sea. He would go much farther than I'd venture to go on my own. Sometimes he'd swim the butterfly stroke with me on his back. I'd try to time my breathing right—inhaling and exhaling, as we moved above and below the water's surface. I was terrified of the idea of going out into the deep water alone, but when I was with my dad, it was different. With him I felt at home in the ocean. He treated the ocean, and all the creatures in it, as if they were part of our family, and over time I learned to do the same.

Everything in my world was going wonderfully, but from my parents' perspective, things weren't quite as carefree. In particular, my dad was struggling with mental health issues. Over the course of a few years my dad's mental state deteriorated greatly. When I was six years old he took his own life, leaving my mom, sister, and me in his wake.

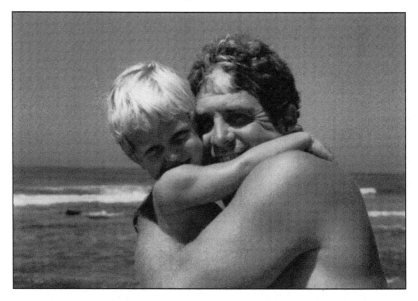

Sebastian and his dad at Windansea Beach. La Jolla, California. Circa 1988

Everything changed after that. The life I had come to know, which was so full of joy, light, and freedom, had been shattered. I felt completely overwhelmed. In the weeks and months following my dad's death I grew more and more closed off. To the best of my ability I blocked off, shut out, and pushed down the sadness, anger, and other emotions that were coming up. This was my plan for survival—I was not going to allow anything or anyone in to hurt me again.

Prior to my dad's death, my mom described me as being incredibly talkative and insatiably curious. I asked about how everything worked and where it all came from. She later told me that after my dad died, my curiosity seemed to have vanished and I hardly spoke. I wouldn't talk about his death, and I shied away from talking about my dad altogether.

Our family dynamic changed as well. Not long after my dad died, we moved out of La Jolla to be closer to my mom's work. She needed to work a lot more to provide for us, and I became more of a caretaker to my younger sister. All of a sudden I had all these new responsibilities. In many ways it felt like that was the end of my childhood.

As I grew older and into my teenage years, I was able to more fully understand what suicide was and the weight of it. I also became more aware of the stigma around it. I didn't talk about my dad or his suicide, but I thought about it constantly. It got to the point where I was struggling greatly with my own mental health. I felt like I was destined to follow in my father's footsteps.

Although much of my childhood was dark after my father died, I was fortunate to have something that probably saved my life: the ocean. Not long after he died, we spread my father's ashes in the ocean at the La Jolla Cove. While the ocean had always been special to me, after he died, it became much more than that; it became my refuge. Whenever I felt sad, lost, or lonely, if I could just get myself down to the beach, my perspective would change. Once I was there, I knew I'd be okay. There, all the vibrancy of life was restored.

I would often think back to when we spread my dad's ashes in the ocean. From that moment on, I saw my father and the ocean as one. Any time I was at the beach or in the ocean, it felt like my dad was right there with me. I saw him in the sand, the water, the seaweed, in the dolphins, fish, and seals swimming by; he was there in every aspect of that wild world.

Going to the beach then became much more than a routine; it became a sacred experience. When I would visit the ocean, everything seemed to slow down. I was present with every step and every breath I took. All my senses became filled with my surroundings. My time at the beach and in the water gave me the strength and determination to keep going back on dry land. I'd return from the ocean renewed and recharged. It was my power source; it was my home. I spent as much time as I could in the ocean. As a result, I became obsessed with body-boarding (aka boogieboarding—similar to surfing, but with a smaller board), and soon my world revolved around the sport.

My experience of living through and learning from my father's suicide became my fuel and passion behind creating Nature Unplugged. My early connection with nature after my dad's suicide has stayed with me and inspired me. It wasn't just having a connection with nature that helped me through the process. There were a number of other lessons learned along the way—the power of mindfulness, human connection, vulnerability—that have become an integral part of this work.

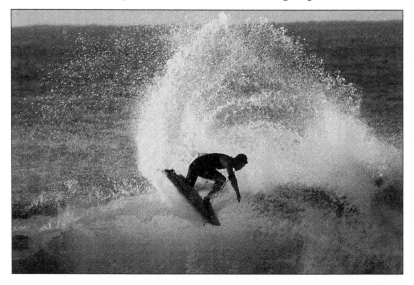

Sebastian on the North Shore of Oahu, Hawaii. Circa 2006. Photo: Keith Laub

My experience has also greatly inspired me to work on suicide prevention and mental health advocacy. I speak regularly on these topics to a wide variety of audiences—K-12 and college students, mental health professionals, educators, and corporate employees. While working with people who are in crisis is deeply important work, I see what we do at Nature Unplugged as being an "upstream" preventive-care approach to mental health. This is really the core of my passion for Nature Unplugged and the work we do. I see this as proactive mental health work to help keep individuals balanced and well so they don't ever need to experience what my dad experienced.

Sonya's Story

I was a cute little monster when I was little. There was a light in me that shone brightly, and my spirit was wild and free. I suffered no confusion over what I liked and what I didn't. I drew on walls, I took things apart that I had no hope or intention of putting back together, I rolled around in the mud and climbed trees, I shouted in grocery stores that I was She-Ra the Princess of Power, and tore through the house like a tornado until I eventually fell asleep sitting upright in a corner. I was hard to handle, no question about that. But there was so much joy and enthusiasm for life radiating from me that I often got a pass from adults to carry on without too much reprimand.

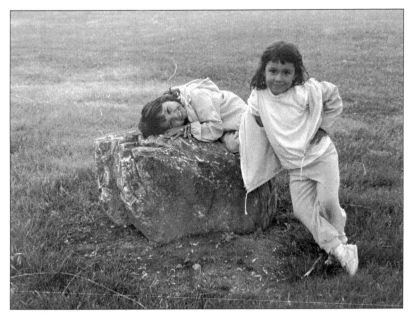

Sonya (right) and her sister (left) in Chesterbrook, PA. Circa 1990

But then things changed, and like most things, they changed slowly over time rather than all of a sudden. I learned that good little girls were quiet when adults told them to be; that you got in trouble if you squirmed in your seat, giggled, or whispered to a friend when the teacher was speaking. I learned that an unpopular opinion was better kept private so as not to offend or upset anyone, and that school was the most important thing in the world—if I didn't do well in school, my future was bleak. Adults rewarded me and granted their approval for improving grades and a high performance in sports; each in their own way improving my odds of going to a good college and setting me on a track to "excel in life." Simultaneously, and often subtly, I was discouraged from pursuing less fruitful endeavors like fine arts, playing outside, and wandering in the nearby forests and parks. Those were less productive, less purposeful activities, with no clear return on a better, brighter future, according to those around me. In fact, they were seen as things that got in the way. They were things I was supposed to grow out of.

I was an average student throughout high school, with some As, some Bs, and a very occasional C. My sister was the academic whiz, not me. I became hyperfocused on soccer and obsessed with playing for a Division I team in college. I played soccer constantly, cross-trained with other sports in high school, and trained at a gym that focused on elevating athletes in their sports. I barely dated, I didn't drink or do drugs, and hardly ever went to parties. I had a goal, and I wasn't interested in compromising my chances of attaining it. Now, I did love the girls on my team and the coaches. I learned a lot about leadership, teamwork, and resilience. Soccer gave me some of my best friends and best memories.

But something changed midway through high school. Something wasn't there that had been previously. I couldn't name it, but I felt its absence, and it created a lot of tension and confusion. I'd go through spells of dreading practice and games. But as soon as I thought about quitting, I quickly dropped the idea. Even the thought made me feel shame and guilt. I had spent too much time and energy already and couldn't even imagine going to college without being a soccer player. What had once been a dream turned into a goal, and all the joy and playfulness melted away. I should be careful here, though, and say that goals are good things, and they certainly don't have to be the death of your dreams. In fact, they're a great way to go after your dreams. But what I didn't realize was that I had become so focused on the goal, the end objective of playing Division I soccer in college, that I had lost myself in it, and it was no longer fun.

I did end up playing Division I soccer. For one year. Then I quit. Then I had a HUGE identity crisis. Who was I without soccer? Shortly after that, my father passed away from pancreatic cancer. He'd had health issues my entire life, but had repeatedly overcome bleak prognosis after bleak prognosis. One part of my brain and heart always knew we were on borrowed time, but the other part thought he was immortal and we'd have him forever. Losing him felt unexpected in many ways. I found myself in what felt like a premature midlife crisis, asking questions like "Who am I?" "What am I doing with my life?" and "What's the point of all this!?"

Social media hadn't emerged yet, and people weren't on their phones constantly. I did have a Super Nintendo console in my dorm room and a tiny TV, but I was fortunate to have a lot of free time and space to reflect, freak out, and try to find myself again. And I started to, slowly. I began reclaiming the pieces of myself that I'd lost touch with. I started to venture back out into nature just for the fun of it. I started to draw and paint again, and even got back into making pottery, which I had enjoyed immensely as a kid. I joined rec sports leagues for fun and played tennis with friends on the community courts. I got involved with clubs on campus and engaged in my community. Who I was had somehow gotten deeply buried in a shell of who I thought I wanted to be, or was supposed to be, and it felt so incredible to be fully alive again.

I have relearned this over and over again, the importance of asking myself what I want, staying in touch with my values and what brings me joy. Because if I lose sight of that, a hundred other people are right there, ready to fill in the blanks for me. That's why I do this work. Because the world around us has gotten so good at selling us their ideas and making us think they're ours. Because there are so many bright, shiny, exciting things vying for our attention that we might never get the chance to discover who we are if we don't make the time and space for it. We are a culture that is overstimulated, overscheduled, oversolicited, and overworked. We have to undo some of that, create some boundaries, and find our way back outside to reclaim our joy, peace, fulfillment, and purpose.

Why the Focus on Technology?

When we founded Nature Unplugged in 2012, the initial vision was about giving people unforgettable experiences in nature, unplugged (without phones and other distracting devices). Our original name was "Experience Nature Unplugged." We led day trips and retreats around Southern California and abroad, incorporating practices like mindfulness, play, and creativity along the way. We offered a variety of guided activities, including hiking, surfing, snorkeling, yoga, and stand-up paddling.

One thing we began to notice early on, especially when working with kids, was how much of a barrier screens and devices were to getting outside and experiencing nature. Apparently video games and media platforms had become a lot cooler and more engaging than when we were kids. We thought getting families and individuals engaged in outdoor activities would be enough to curb the pull of technology and create more balance. For some of our clients, that was true, but for the majority of them, the pull of technology was stronger than the pull of nature.

As this trend became more apparent to us, we began to focus our attention on what this was all about. It was around that time that we started to read the growing body of research about the impact of technology on our attention and our well-being. We also began to more formally explore the research about the benefits of nature and how nature can act as an antidote to technology overuse.

In 2015, we had the opportunity to do a deeper dive on this. We began a graduate program studying leadership at the University of San Diego. In addition to our studies of leadership theory and practice, organizational psychology, and group dynamics, we focused our research and thesis on how increased screen time and technology impacts one's capacity for leadership.

We were particularly interested in learning how an increase in tech use affected skills often used in the practice of leadership. Things like face-to-face communication, eye contact, teamwork, empathy for others, feeling emotions, the ability to hold off on short-term gratification for the long-term goal of the group, to name a few. Based on our experiences, we assumed that increased tech use would be causing the most significant issues with iGen (born after 1995, iGen—aka Generation Z—is the first generation to spend their entire adolescence in the age of the smartphone), which wasn't entirely true. The dramatic increase of tech use that accompanied the rise of smartphones in 2011 has impacted us all (albeit in different ways), from iGen to Millennials to Boomers.

How to Use This Book

At Nature Unplugged, our methodology is based on research, our field work with clients, and our own personal experiences. Our approach is a holistic one. We offer a combination of technical solutions that can be implemented right away and other work that requires deep reflection, time, and commitment. There are no magic bullets here. For some, this book will simply plant the seeds of change. It could take some time for the ideas to take hold and inspire the necessary motivation to fully embark on this journey. For most folks, and hopefully you, you're ready to break free from the clutches of technology overuse, reconnect with nature, and engage with life and work in a whole new way. Something has felt off, and it's time to make some moves, which is why you got this book.

THE EXPERIENCE NATURE UNPLUGGED (ENU) METHOD

The structure of this book is based on how we work with clients. It is divided into five parts that build on each other and are the essential steps in the ENU Method: Reframe, Reset, Reconnect, Rewire, and Recharge. This process is a pathway that helps us navigate a noisy world full of distractions, competing priorities, and endless to-do lists. Here's a quick overview of the ENU Method, which will guide us on our journey toward wellness in the digital age.

PART I: REFRAME

First things first—we need to explore and examine the challenges of living in the digital age. Why do we have such a hard time putting down our phones? Where has all our free time gone? How are we using technology and digital media in our day-to-day lives? And, where is it benefiting us and where is it getting in the way? Finding balance and wellness today requires us to understand what the digital age is and how the attention economy (the immense pull of social media and tech in our lives) works. There's a lot happening behind the scenes that keeps us glued to our devices. By the end of Part I, we'll understand the challenges of living in the digital age (the problem we're addressing), which is foundational to reframing how we approach and manage our relationship with technology.

PART II: RESET

While it's important to understand the problem we're facing, this book is really about stepping into the solutions. We like to think of pushing a big red reset button here. This is all about becoming more intentional with our tech and bringing more nature into our lives. We'll introduce our "Four Steps to Reset" process, which helps redefine our relationship with tech and nature. By using boundaries to minimize our daily digital distractions, we open up space in our day to include more time in nature unplugged. Nature is one of the greatest antidotes to technology overuse. In a high-tech world, we need higher doses of nature time to restore the balance. By the end of Part II, we'll emerge from our media haze and be able to focus on what's important.

PART III: RECONNECT

This part of the journey addresses two of the biggest challenges of tech overuse: an increasingly sedentary lifestyle and isolation. Modern technology offers comfort, convenience, and the ability to be connected 24/7. Yet as a society we're sitting more, moving less, and we are more isolated and alone than at any other time in our history. As a result, we're suffering physically and mentally. To address this, we'll focus on the importance of movement and how to bring more community and connection into our lives. By the end of Part III, we'll have reconnected to our bodies and each other.

PART IV: REWIRE

It may be helpful to think of the earlier parts as the tangible fixes that set us on the right path and get us out of our own way. We call them technical solutions. If "Reset" and "Reconnect" are the tip of the iceberg, then "Rewire" is about diving beneath the surface and doing the deeper and more adaptive work. This part is all about building and strengthening your inner force field against the attention economy. Doing this inner work opens us up to new possibilities and will help ensure that we don't get pulled back into old patterns. By the end of Part IV, we will have rewired how we think, approach challenges, deal with disappointment, celebrate successes, and cultivate curiosity.

PART V: RECHARGE

This work is not about just getting to a baseline; it's about getting in touch with what we want and stepping into our potential. We're ready to explore, adventure, try new things, and engage with life and the world around us in a completely new way. Here we'll look at how to recharge our batteries through the power of play and by bringing more creativity into our lives. By the end of this part, and the end of this book, we will have decluttered our digital lives, reconnected with ourselves, each other, and the world around us. We'll have moved from surviving to thriving.

~

The chapters within each part will zoom in and provide a combination of research and personal stories as well as practical tips and tools for you to put what you've learned into action right away. To help with that, there will be a series of exercises at the end of each chapter. While it may be tempting to skip them, we highly recommend taking the time to complete each one. Of course, it's entirely up to you. As we share with our coaching clients, the energy you put into this process will directly translate to what you get out of it. For those looking for more exercises and resources, check out https://www.natureunplugged.com. There you'll find additional tips, tools, and resources to help support your journey of wellness in the digital age.

Following is a visual representation of the ENU Method. When beginning this work, it's important that we work our way through each part in the order presented. Each piece builds on the one before and will help prepare us as we make our way through the process.

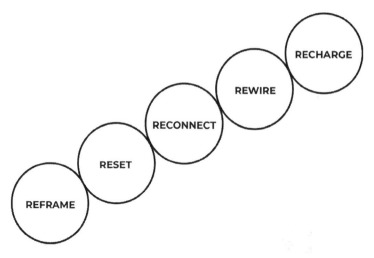

While it's helpful to see each step laid out in a step-by-step order initially, the reality is that it's more of a dynamic process. Once we get the basics of each part down, we will continue to work with all of the parts as we grow and develop.

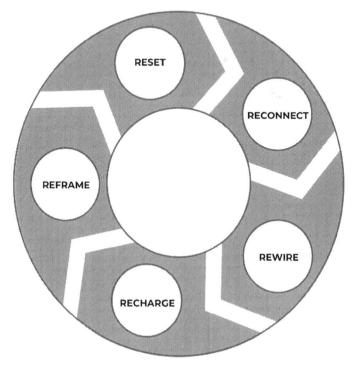

Philosophy and Contract

At the end of this book you will have the opportunity to create your own personal philosophy for wellness in the digital age and complete an ENU contract. We've found these tools to be highly effective in our coaching work. While having the knowledge of what to do is important, the key is being able to put that knowledge into practice. The philosophy and contract are designed to help you do just that.

Your philosophy for wellness in the digital age is a short (one- or two-paragraph) statement that helps guide your path moving forward. It helps give you the 30,000-foot view and the bigger picture. Your contract, on the other hand, offers more concrete and actionable ways to put your philosophy to work in your day-to-day life. The two combined are powerful tools that will support you in your pursuit of wellness in the digital age. When you're feeling uncertain about your path, return to this philosophy and contract to help guide your decisions so that they align with your values.

Activity: Setting Your Intention

Now that you have a sense of what's to come over the course of this book, we're excited to get going! However, we have one final disclaimer before moving on to the first part of the ENU Method. The research, tips, and tools in the pages to come are incredible resources in this journey. But an intellectual understanding of these concepts will only get you so far. The key is putting this knowledge into practice. Our role is to help guide, motivate, and challenge you. But, we won't be doing the work for you. How you engage with the content and utilize this book is entirely up to you. While there is no right or wrong, it is important to be intentional. By the end of this book, what do you want to have changed? What's your motivation for reading this book? What do you hope to get out of it? Before moving on, let's lay the foundation for this work and take a moment to explore and reflect on your motivation and goals.

Take some time to think about what you want to get out of this and write it below. Clarifying your purpose and setting an intention will help you to stay focused and energized. When you find that you're distracted or unmotivated, return to your intention to remind yourself of why you're doing this in the first place. **Be honest. Be specific. Be as personal and real as possible.**

MY INTENTION: _____

_____

_____

_____

_____

_____

_____

_____

_____

_____

_____

_____

_____

_____

_____

_____

_____

_____

_____

PAUSE AND REFLECT

The practice of reflection allows us to sort through ideas and examine a variety of possibilities and options. Throughout this book, we will offer space to clarify your thoughts, find answers, and understand what questions remain. There's no specific amount of time required—take as little or as much time as you need to consider the questions posed.

- *What does a healthy relationship with technology look like to you?*
- *What does a healthy relationship with nature look like to you?*

INTRODUCTION

PART ONE

REFRAME

How to Change the Way We Think about Technology and Digital Media

To begin, we will explore and examine the challenges of living in the digital age. Why do we have such a hard time putting down our phones? Where has all our free time gone? How are we using technology in our day-to-day lives? And, where is it benefiting us and where is it getting in the way? Finding balance and wellness today requires us to understand what the digital age is and how the attention economy (the immense pull of social media and tech in our lives) works. There's a lot happening behind the scenes that keeps us glued to our devices. By the end of Part I, we'll understand the challenges of living in the digital age (the problem we're addressing), which is foundational to reframing how we approach and manage our relationship with technology.

CHAPTER 1

Challenges of Living in the Digital Age

— ♪ —

The average person checks their phone 150 times a day.
Why do we do this?
Are we making 150 conscious choices?
—Tristan Harris

A useful place to begin is by examining the challenges of living in the digital age. Here we'll explore the impact on our brains, bodies, and lives of being overconnected to technology and disconnected from nature. It's critical to have a clear understanding of the situation—to fully know what you're up against—in order to find the solutions that will work best for you.

Before diving headfirst into the problem, let's step back for a moment and focus on the bigger picture. We opened this book with a simple yet powerful question: What's the most valuable nonrenewable resource we have? The answer, of course, is our time. We don't know how much time we have here. And, knowing our time is finite, how are we going to spend it?

When we consider the concept of time and how we're spending it, we often think of a good friend of ours, Mark Kalina, who is a doctor. He's not just any doctor. He's an incredible one. Throughout his career he's been at the forefront of the movement toward more holistic and integrative primary care, and he now works at Pacific Pearl in La Jolla, California—an integrative medical practice and wellness center. He cares deeply for his patients, and that shines through in every aspect of his work. In addition to primary care, for the past twenty years he's worked a great deal with hospice patients. He helps his patients and their families have the best end-of-life experience possible.

In his hospice work, Dr. Kalina takes care of any medical needs his patients may have. In addition to the medical and technical needs, he's also there to listen to and comfort his patients, right up until the end of their lives. They have an opportunity to share whatever they want to share. Dr. Kalina tells us these are often their most profound memories, loves, losses, lessons and insights. They aren't reflecting on their social media presence, number of followers, funny memes or videos, or apps they fondly remember. They share deep experiences that are rooted in connection to themselves, each other, and the world around them, just as most of us would at such a time. You can imagine how powerful and real these conversations are. There is no time or room for anything else.

We're sharing Dr. Kalina's experience because it's a hugely important reminder that we don't have an unlimited amount of time on Earth. We've known Dr. Kalina for the past ten years and this is a topic we talk about often. And, over the course of our relationship with Dr. Kalina, contemplating the end of life has become a regular practice for us. When we think about this, we wonder what we would want to talk about in our final days. When we look back, what will be the most important and meaningful lessons?

Imagine you're at the end of your life and you have the opportunity to share your most meaningful memories and lessons. What would they be? Would you speak about time spent with family, friends, and loved ones? Would your thoughts center on big and exciting adventures and trips? Would you smile and share the little things, the mannerisms and quirks of people close to you, or the sounds of the birds on a spring morning as you sipped coffee on your front porch?

Regardless of how old you are or how much time you think you have to live, this is a powerful practice. It brings perspective to how we spend our time and clarity on what's truly important. That clarity and perspective provide important context for how we frame the challenges of living in the digital age. We know we have a limited amount of time here. Yet, many of us spend much of our precious time glued to our devices. Specifically, this becomes a problem when our tech use isn't conscious or intentional.

The pull to use our devices more often and stay on them longer can feel overpowering and intense. And it's not you, it's the tech; the technology—the devices, the applications, the algorithms, the software—is strong and clever. It's designed to grab your attention and hold it for as long as possible. Even the sound of a notification—a new message, incoming email, news alert or "like"—has become a dopamine feedback loop that makes us want to hear it again and again. The rise of smart technology has brought with it incredible benefits and conveniences. However, those benefits come with drawbacks. In certain ways we are more connected than ever before, yet we are increasingly disconnected from ourselves, each other, and the world around us.

Challenges of Living in the Digital Age

The impact of technology use and screen time on our mental and physical well-being is real and the research is mounting. There's a lot of information out there (an overwhelming amount!) and our aim is to break it down and give you a clearer picture of what we're dealing with. With that said, this is by no means an exhaustive dive into research. Once you have a basic understanding of the problem—the negative impact of unmitigated tech use, the attention economy, and the fact that technology is no longer neutral—you don't need to go much further (unless you really want to).

It's also important to acknowledge that the research landscape around technology and digital media use is constantly changing, and doing so at a rapid pace. In addition to combing through studies and research for this book, we had the opportunity to interview a number of top researchers and experts in the field. One of those experts is Dr. Larry Rosen, a research psychologist from California State University, Dominguez Hills, who is recognized as an international expert in the psychology of technology. Dr. Rosen shared with us just how quickly this world is changing. As an example, he told us about a class he teaches on the global impact of technology. When the class begins he hands out his syllabus and states, "Here's my syllabus, but don't believe it. Because something is going to happen over the course of this semester—the release of a new social media app or piece of smart technology—that is going to change the focus of the class."

For similar reasons, we're not going to do a deep dive into the current trends of big social media platforms like Facebook, Instagram, and Snapchat in this book. By the time you read this, it's entirely possible that a new app or social media platform will emerge that changes our behavior and culture. Instead, we'll spend time looking at the foundational and relatively evergreen aspects of the issues with technology that will remain relevant in the years to come.

As we lay out the challenges of living in this digital age, including some of the latest research about technology and screen time, remember that our intention isn't to scare you into changing your relationship with technology. It's to give you a basic understanding of the problem so that we can work together toward solutions that work and fit your life. So, let's get going.

In a nutshell, the problem we are addressing is that we are over-connected to technology and we are disconnected from nature. Richard Louv—author of *Last Child in the Woods* and the inspiration for an international movement to reconnect children to nature—is a huge inspiration to us at Nature Unplugged. Louv coined the term "Nature Deficit Disorder," which is used to describe the effect of human alienation from nature and the resulting behavioral problems. The combination of our nature deficit and technology overuse contributes to many negative outcomes relating to our mental and physical health and well-being. We're seeing higher instances of attention disorders, anxiety, depression, isolation, and suicide. Some of the physical ailments that come with more sedentary lifestyles include high blood pressure, diabetes, and obesity.

Collectively, we tend to point our fingers at younger generations when we think about this issue. The reality is, it's affecting people regardless of their age, gender, race, or socioeconomic status. Take a look at these statistics to get a better picture of the situation.

TECHNOLOGY USE—KIDS
- Smartphone ownership has grown substantially between 2015 and 2019.
  - Nearly one in five (19%) 8-year-olds have their own smartphone.
  - By age 11, a majority (53%) of kids have their own smartphone.
  - By age 12, more than two-thirds (69%) do.
  - 84% of 13- to 18-year-olds own a smartphone.[10]

- On average, 8- to 12-year-olds in the U.S. use around 4.5 hours of entertainment screen media per day (4:44), and teens use around 7.5 hours—not including time spent using screens for school or homework.[11]
- Half of teenagers say they "feel addicted" to their mobile device and 72% say they feel the need to immediately respond to texts and social networking messages.[12]

TECHNOLOGY USE—ADULTS

- 96% of adults own a cell phone and 81% own smartphones in the United States.[13]
- 81% of Americans say they go online on a daily basis.[14]
- Roughly 3-in-10 US adults report they are "almost constantly" online.[15]

IMPACT OF TECHNOLOGY USE ON SLEEP

- Children who use a media device right before bed are:
  - More likely to sleep less than they should, more likely to sleep poorly, and more than twice as likely to be sleepy during the day.[16]
  - Sleep deprivation is linked to compromised thinking and reasoning, susceptibility to illness, weight gain, and high blood pressure. It also affects mood: People who don't sleep enough are prone to depression and anxiety.[17]
- Problematic internet use and internet gaming are associated with poor sleep, and researchers believe the high correlation between internet use and depression may stem from difficulty sleeping.[18]
- Excessive computer use during leisure time is associated with sleep problems in adults working a regular daytime schedule.[19]
- Use of computers and mobile phones in the bedroom are related to poor sleep habits and symptoms of insomnia in adults.[20]
- Bedtime mobile phone use is negatively related to sleep outcomes in adults, worse sleep efficiency, more sleep disturbance, and shorter sleep duration.[21]

IMPACT OF TECHNOLOGY USE ON MENTAL HEALTH

- A study of 3,000 children and adolescents followed over three years found that youth who spent more time playing video games were more impulsive and had more attention problems.[22]
- Excessive internet use in children and adolescents is linked to impairment in thoughts and feelings, difficulty making friends, and lowered school performance.[23]
- Teens who spend three hours a day or more on electronic devices are 35% more likely to have a risk factor for suicide, such as making a suicide plan.[24]
- A study of young adults (19–32 years old) found that people with higher social media use were more than three times as likely to feel socially isolated than those who did not use social media as often.[25]

DIRECT AND INDIRECT IMPACT OF TECHNOLOGY USE ON PHYSICAL HEALTH

- The majority of adults (81.6%) and adolescents (81.8%) do not get the recommended amount of physical activity.[26]
- One in four Americans, or 81.2 million people, age six and older are physically inactive.[27]
- Data from 2017–2018 indicates that 42.4% of U.S. adults were obese.[28]
- Data from 2015–2016 indicates that 13.9% of children ages 2–5 years old, 18.4% of children ages 6–11 years old, and 20.6% of children ages 12–19 years old are obese in the U.S.[29]
- A five-year study found an association between texting on a mobile phone and neck or upper back pain in young adults.[30]

Is Technology Neutral?

The purpose of this list isn't to freak you out. The point is to illustrate that we are living in a time when we are extremely attached to and dependent on our smart technology. Our relationships with devices have changed dramatically since 2012 (when smartphones became widely accessible). It's important to call that out, understand it, and examine it. One thing we often hear in response to the rise of these negative outcomes is, "Well, that's because people are overusing tech nowadays.

Technology is like a tool, it's neutral. You use it when you want to and put it down when you don't." And at first, that response is easy to accept as it sounds very logical; but unfortunately, it's not that simple.

What makes this so challenging and what makes our relationship with technology complicated is that it is no longer neutral. When we say technology, we're referring to high-tech, smart devices like smartphones, tablets, computers, TVs, and wearable technology. Old landline phones, your microwave, and vacuum cleaner are good examples of technology that is low-tech and neutral (although this keeps changing too, like smart fridges, for example). The point is, folks are typically in control of when they're vacuuming or reheating their food. One of the big differences is that our high-tech, smart devices are web-enabled tools that connect us to a variety of digital media, software, and apps. Behind every app, software, and platform there are tons of intelligent people (many of whom have studied psychology and neuroscience) designing technology and programs to overpower and undermine our willpower. That's why leaving your favorite app or putting down your phone can seem so hard.

It's important to highlight and understand the role dopamine plays in all of this. Trevor Haynes, a research technician in the Department of Neurobiology at Harvard Medical School, wrote an article in 2018 that helps explain how dopamine and technology and digital media interact.[31] Dopamine, Haynes explains, is a chemical produced by our brains that plays a starring role in motivating behavior. When we take a bite of delicious food, have sex, exercise, and, importantly, when we have successful social interactions, dopamine is released in our bodies. It's the body's way of rewarding us for beneficial behaviors and motivates us to repeat them. Similarly, positive social stimuli—laughing faces, positive reinforcement and recognition by our peers, messages from loved ones—results in a release of dopamine, reinforcing whatever behavior came before it. Haynes continues by highlighting that smartphones have provided us with an unending supply of social stimuli, both positive and negative. Every notification has the potential to produce a dopamine hit, which is why we check our phones hundreds of times a day.

People like former Google programmer Tristan Harris have been doing wonderful work in recent years to expose these types of practices. Here are a few common examples of how technology undermines our willpower.

SCROLLING FEEDS

If you've spent time on Facebook or Instagram (or any other social media and news platform), you'll notice that there's a continuous scroll of information, updates, and news to explore. Typically these scrolls never end, and you could spend hours scrolling away without leaving the page you're on. Remember how we used to scroll to the bottom of a webpage and then have to click "next page" to see more? There are no more natural pauses that allow or encourage conscious thought. Previously, when the page ended, there was space to ask ourselves if we had found what we were looking for or if we wanted to continue searching and scrolling. It forced us to make and remake decisions to stay or leave. This new clever design keeps us scrolling and engaged on platforms longer, with few, if any, pauses or prompts to consider whether we'd like to stop or keep going.

AUTOPLAY

This is another ingenious design. Autoplay is the feature that's often preset on video platforms like YouTube and Netflix. This design feature automatically queues and plays the next episode or video with related content (news story, dancing kitten, sports replay, etc.) within a few seconds. You've probably seen this before, but have you thought about its impact? You're enjoying a relaxing evening watching one of your favorite shows on Netflix. You're getting sleepy and plan on going to bed after the current episode ends. But before you can make any moves to get up off the couch and head to your bedroom, a little timer shows up on your screen giving you five seconds before automatically starting the next episode. Alas, you were too slow to stop it, and the next episode has begun. You're quickly pulled back in and find yourself settling back into the couch for one last episode. This cycle can, and often does, repeat itself into the wee hours of the night.

SNAPSTREAKS

Gamification, the process of gamelike elements to encourage participation, is another way to keep people using social media platforms, like Snapchat, more often and longer. A Snapstreak is when you and a friend exchange at least one snap (aka message) per day for several consecutive days. Once you begin your streak, you get little prizes and emojis as you build up your streak and hit certain benchmarks like five days or a hundred days. This is a simple and highly effective way to gamify messaging. At the same time, it's also creating an informal way to measure and rate how close friendships are. The longer your streak is, the "better and closer" the friendship is. The fact that this measure is arbitrary doesn't matter. It feels real and it feels important. Many users experience immense social pressure to keep Snapstreaks going, and that's exactly what the programmers aimed to achieve. The more social pressure, the more likely users will feel pushed to maintain their streaks.

Honestly, we didn't quite grasp the power of Snapstreaks until one of our Nature Unplugged retreats a few years back. We host regular retreats, and this particular retreat was with college-age students. These are three-day "Digital Detox" retreats, offering space to unplug and focus on hiking, exploring, connecting with nature, and practicing mindfulness.

In 2016, around the time when Snapstreaks first came out, we were packing up and about to head out on a guided nature retreat when we noticed a huge amount of distress coming from students about being away from their phones. It's typical for students to worry about leaving their phones (and other devices) behind, but this anxiety was on another level. We had several anxious students approach us before getting in the group van to see if we would make an exception and give them access to their phones during the retreat. After asking the students what was going on, we found out that the spike in anxiety was over losing their Snapstreaks, some of which had spanned many months and were highly valued in their friendships. A couple of days after that trip, we found out that some students made elaborate plans to give their phones and passwords to friends so that they could keep their Snapstreaks intact while they were away. This was a real eye-opener for us. It demonstrated how intense the social pressure can be and how effective some of these tactics are in keeping people engaged with social media platforms.

.

~

Scrolling feeds, autoplay, and Snapstreaks exemplify how back-end designs by developers can change how we engage with our devices. The way these platforms grab and keep our attention means our devices are no longer neutral. And because our smart devices aren't neutral, it's our responsibility to be vigilant and aware of these tactics. The greater our awareness, the more power we have to be intentional in using our technology. And that's the goal: to rise above the digital noise and distraction and use technology intentionally, in ways that serve and benefit us. More on that to come!

The Attention Economy

Understanding that technology isn't neutral helps us make sense of how the attention economy has changed our relationships with technology. The quote by Tristan Harris at the beginning of this chapter exemplifies how the attention economy affects us. "The average person checks their phone 150 times a day. Why do we do this? Are we making 150 conscious choices?" No. Of course we're not making those choices consciously. In fact, it's so deeply unconscious, it doesn't even feel like a choice.

So, how does the attention economy work? What is it? The business model is simple. The more user attention a platform can get, the more effective its advertising space becomes. The more effective the advertising space becomes, the more a platform can charge advertisers. We often think about the currency of our economy in terms of dollars. This economy is similar, but the currency is our attention. All day every day, tech companies of all sizes are vying for our attention. They are doing whatever they can to keep us on their platform, website, game, or app for as long as they can. Because the longer they have our attention, the more opportunity they have to earn advertising revenue.

When using platforms like Facebook, Instagram, and Snapchat, it's critical to understand that we, the users, are not the customers. We are the product being sold to companies so they can advertise effectively and directly to us. Data on our search terms, browsing habits, media use, and post engagement are continuously captured and stored, creating a rich advertising profile for each of us. In 2020, Facebook reported having nine million active advertisers using their social networking platform to promote their products and services.[32] Facebook generates almost all of its revenue through advertising, which amounted to 69.7 billion U.S. dollars in 2019.[33] The bottom line for these companies is to get our attention and to hold on to it regardless of how that impacts us as people. This is also directly connected to technology not being neutral.

Sebastian's Story: My First Smartphone

I remember getting my first smartphone. It was an iPhone, and I was an undergrad at the time. Like many other people, I was blown away by how amazing and multifunctional it was. All of a sudden I had access to so much information, and endless features and tools were at my fingertips. In addition to calls and texts, I could listen to music, browse the internet, and check my email. It was incredible. As the years passed and updated versions came out, I didn't think twice about upgrading to the latest technology. I wanted access to more tools and widgets, advanced features, and increased functionality.

Initially, I was quite intentional about what I wanted on my smartphone, but over time that faded as I got caught up in the novelty of having the latest and greatest that tech could offer. The problem was that as time went on, I found myself overconnected and overwhelmed with too many apps, emails, and notifications. In a sneaky ninja-like way, tech companies had convinced me that the most important thing was to always have the newest technology, regardless of what it was, whether I was enjoying it, or if it was serving me or my goals.

It was similar to when I signed up for my first social media account on Myspace back in the early 2000s. (Remember Myspace?) Initially it was a really neat thing. I didn't use Myspace a whole lot, but when I did, it was a great tool. I was traveling extensively at the time and it was a way for me to stay connected with friends all over the world and to get a sense of what they were up to. Myspace came and went, and then Facebook appeared. The original Facebook was similar to Myspace, and it was a useful tool to stay connected with family and friends all over the world.

Over the years, the platform evolved and things started to shift. As the platform changed, so did my relationship with it. My level of engagement and time spent on Facebook skyrocketed. More features were added: the Like button, the Poke, the endless newsfeed scroll, messaging, calls, and live stories. At some point, Facebook went from being something I used intentionally every once in a while to connect with friends and family to something I logged into every day, multiple times a day. It became a virtual hangout spot, something to do when I was bored or had some downtime. Eventually, checking my social media feed was an unconscious habit. I'd be waiting in line at the grocery store, on an elevator, in the bathroom, or procrastinating on homework, and find myself scrolling through Facebook without any purpose or reason. Later, other platforms like Instagram, Snapchat, and TikTok joined the scene and brought things to a whole new level.

There was always something new and exciting to check out, so it was (and is) hard not to get swept up in it. Rarely did I take the time to think, *Hmmm, do I really want the latest version of Angry Birds on my phone? Do I want access to emails 24/7? Do I want continuous push notifications from various social media and news platforms throughout the day? Are these things adding value to my life or are they a distraction?* I suspect I'm not alone in that experience. Somewhere along the way, these amazing, novel, unobtrusive platforms and technologies transformed into pervasive and aggressive entities in our lives. They became Godzilla-like tech monsters rampaging around, doing everything they could to gain and keep our attention (maybe too extreme a metaphor, but you get the picture).

Of course, it's important to point out that it's not all bad. There are some really awesome and valuable aspects to smart devices and technology. We love having the ability to take photos on our phones without having to lug around a camera. Being able to video chat with family and friends in far-off places is incredible. Access to education and information is amazing. As we have stated before, this isn't about being anti-tech. The balance is what's important. Being intentional about what technology we use and how we use it is the key.

What Tech Leaders Do

If you were a fly on the wall in the homes of some of the bigwig leaders in the tech industry, you might be surprised by what you find. How do the people who have led the way in creating our smart devices, software, and applications use them in their daily lives? You might imagine that these Silicon Valley techies (and their families) are using their devices nonstop, and that their children are swimming in tech from a very young age. It turns out to be just the opposite. Leaders in tech often have strict rules and boundaries with their own technology use and that of their families. Numerous articles and interviews over the past ten years have highlighted this. Most notably, Bill Gates of Microsoft didn't let his kids have cell phones until they were 14 years old. Steve Jobs of Apple didn't let his kids use iPads and significantly limited his kids' device use at home.[34] And, Evan Spiegel of Snapchat limited his children to 1.5 hours of screen time per week.[35]

In a 2011 article from the *New York Times* titled "A Silicon Valley School That Doesn't Compute," Matt Richtel describes how many of the children of tech leaders in Silicon Valley grow up attending Waldorf schools.[36] These schools differ from a typical public education in many ways, but most notably, they are almost completely tech-free. They don't use computers and they don't use screens. Instead, students learn through creativity, physical activity, and hands-on projects. Instead of computers and other high-tech devices, they use analog materials and spend a lot of time engaging in nature. It's fascinating to see that the vast majority of schools across the country are full of computers and tablets and other devices, while many of the children of those who created these devices are learning the old-fashioned way.

These tech leaders are being very intentional about their use of technology because they know the impact tech overuse has on our well-being. And this intentionality is at the core of our philosophy on technology.

What's Your Daily Tech Diet?

In order for us to improve our relationship with technology, using it more intentionally, we have to critically examine how we're currently using it. Remember, it's not about what's right or wrong in terms of tech and media use. It certainly isn't about shaming or blaming either. The point here is to raise our level of awareness and feel empowered in the choices we're making. Bringing awareness to how our time is spent each day is a critical first step. Once we know how frequently we engage with technology, and what type of technology we use, we can begin cultivating a healthier relationship with technology that promotes balance and intention. Instead of unconsciously surfing the web or endlessly scrolling social media feeds, we embrace and acknowledge that we have a choice.

Activity: Time and Tech Use

Take a moment to reflect on how you are spending your time each day, with particular attention to your use of technology and digital media. From there you can explore how your tech use helps or hinders you from achieving your goals and moving forward with purpose.

Excluding your technology and digital media use for work or school, use this exercise to figure out what your tech and media diet is. Check all media types that apply and estimate how much time (hrs/mins) you spend by category on a typical weekday. Add your totals by category to find your daily total.

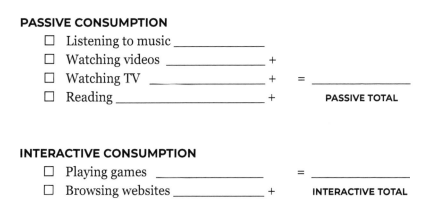

PASSIVE CONSUMPTION
- ☐ Listening to music _____
- ☐ Watching videos _____ +
- ☐ Watching TV _____ + = _____
- ☐ Reading _____ + **PASSIVE TOTAL**

INTERACTIVE CONSUMPTION
- ☐ Playing games _____ = _____
- ☐ Browsing websites _____ + **INTERACTIVE TOTAL**

CREATION

- ☐ Making digital art _____
- ☐ Composing music _____ +
- ☐ Writing _____ +   = _____
- ☐ Programming _____ +   **CREATION TOTAL**

COMMUNICATION

- ☐ Using social media _____   = _____
- ☐ Calls and messaging _____ +   **COMM. TOTAL**

_____ + _____ + _____ + _____ = _____

| PASSIVE TOTAL | INTERACTIVE TOTAL | CREATION TOTAL | COMM. TOTAL | DAILY MEDIA TOTAL |

Now you have an estimate of how much time you spend with technology on a typical day, and a sense of how you use technology during that time. Use the plate that follows to visually represent this. Reference the example on the following page as a guide.

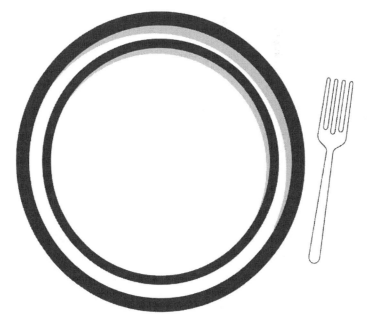

EXAMPLE

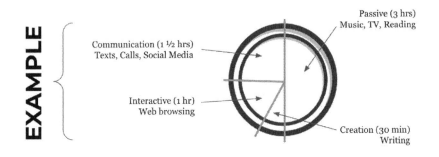

Communication (1 ½ hrs)
Texts, Calls, Social Media

Interactive (1 hr)
Web browsing

Passive (3 hrs)
Music, TV, Reading

Creation (30 min)
Writing

PAUSE AND REFLECT

- *What aspects of technology do you appreciate the most, and why? (In other words, what is most helpful? What do you get the most enjoyment out of?)*
- *What aspects of technology do you appreciate the least, and why? (In other words, what gets in the way? What is most problematic for you?)*

TIME MAPPING

How do you spend your time? The circle below represents a 24-hour day broken into four quarters. Map out how you spend your time on a typical day. Make this as detailed as you can, including as many activities as you can think of (i.e., sleeping, time at work or school, preparing or eating meals, watching TV, time in nature, sports, exercise, relaxing). That way you'll get an accurate picture. You may find it helpful to pick the most recent weekday to model this after.

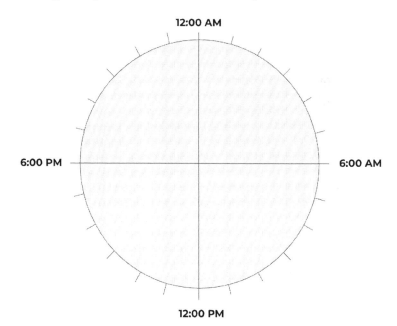

12:00 AM

6:00 PM

6:00 AM

12:00 PM

PAUSE AND REFLECT

- *What do you notice about your 24-hour time map?*
- *Did anything surprise you?*
- *Are there activities you'd like to be doing more of?*
- *If so, what are they?*
- *What could you do less of to free up time in your day?*

Time is our most valuable nonrenewable resource. Fast-forward and imagine that you're at the end of your life. You have an opportunity for one last moment of reflection. What are your fondest memories? What have been your biggest takeaways?

Now, come back to the present. How does what you wrote impact your relationship with technology?

NOTES:_____

_____

_____

_____

_____

_____

_____

_____

_____

_____

_____

_____

_____

_____

_____

_____

_____

_____

_____

CHAPTER 2

Leadership in the Digital Age

꒱

*If you find that what you do each day
seems to have no link to any higher purpose, you probably
want to rethink what you're doing.*
—Ronald A. Heifetz

As we mentioned in the Introduction, while in our Leadership Studies graduate program at the University of San Diego we had the opportunity to research and examine the impact technology overuse and time in nature has on well-being. Specifically, we wanted to know how the practice of leadership was affected by the rise of screen time. Based on our experiences, we assumed that increased tech use would specifically and disproportionately impact young people. While there are significant effects among youth, we were surprised to find that the issues that arise from increased tech use and decreased time spent in nature impact everyone significantly—iGen, Millennials, Generation X, and Boomers.

Needless to say, we came away from our graduate program with a shift in perspective. In addition to viewing the challenges of living in the digital age as a health and wellness issue, we began to see this as a leadership issue. There is a tremendous and emerging need for leadership among individuals, families, and communities in this arena. Be warned, though: stepping up to this call is not for the faint of heart. As we will learn, the practice of leadership is often challenging and comes with a cost.

Looking at the challenges of living in the digital age through the lens of leadership frames our approach and offers a foundation for the solutions we'll offer. While the connection to leadership may not seem obvious yet, it will soon. Whether you're a parent interested in bringing more balance and well-being to yourself and your family, a professional looking to help your team at work (or both), or an individual interested in your own personal development, the practice of leadership is required to do this work effectively and meaningfully.

What Is Leadership?

Leadership is a broad topic, and there are countless definitions, views, and philosophies out there. The way we talk about leadership may be different from what you're used to. To clarify and make sure we're on the same page, here's our view of leadership (in short): *The leader you are is the person you are. Leadership is not a noun, a position you hold, or a set of traits. It happens from the inside out. To exercise leadership requires self-awareness, courage, clear values and vision, and the ability for self-compassion and care.* This is our way of talking about leadership and is foundational to the rest of the book.

ADAPTIVE LEADERSHIP

Early on in our graduate studies, we were introduced to the framework of Adaptive Leadership, and it has been central to our work ever since. It helped us see the issue of increased technology use and disconnection from nature as an adaptive challenge as well as a technical problem. The Adaptive Leadership framework was codeveloped by Ronald Heifetz and Marty Linsky at the Center for Public Leadership at Harvard Kennedy School. Heifetz and Linsky define Adaptive Leadership as the practice of mobilizing people to face tough challenges and thrive.

A central tenet of Adaptive Leadership is this: before trying to solve a problem, it's important to understand and identify what type of problem you're facing. From Ronald Heifetz's perspective, "the single biggest failure of leadership is to treat adaptive challenges like technical problems."

So what's the difference between the two?

Technical Problem: An example of a technical problem is a broken arm. When you break your arm, it's easy to identify what the issue is. You know what you need to do (go to the hospital), and who will help you fix it (a doctor). There is a fairly straightforward and known solution for this problem, including the recovery time and process. Technical problems are easy to identify, can often be solved by an expert in the field, and solutions can typically be implemented quickly.

Adaptive Challenge: When you have a heart attack, it's a little more complicated. The first step is similar, in that you'll need to get emergency care and be treated by a doctor. The doctor, the expert, will do what needs to be done to restore the functioning of your heart. That may include inserting a stent to open a blocked passageway or a different intervention. That part is technical, but what comes after that is adaptive work. To reduce the chance of it happening again, you'll have to make some big changes. You'll need to change your lifestyle (what you eat, how often you exercise, minimize stress), and other people will be involved (your family, friends, coworkers, other health and medical specialists, etc.). With an adaptive challenge, the solution is more difficult to identify and achieve. While there are experts who can recommend what to do, the solution that has worked for others may not work for you. There are many variables at play, and finding a solution will require some trial and error and experimentation.

The following chart is adapted from Heifitz and Linsky's work and illustrates the difference between adaptive and technical challenges:

TECHNICAL	ADAPTIVE
Easy to identify; Known	Difficult to identify; Unknown
Typically have quick and easy solutions	Solutions take time and can be complex
Can turn to authority figures or experts for solutions	People with the problem do the work of solving it
Change required is often specific, clear and generally isolated in one area	Change required can be ambiguous and cross multiple areas
People are generally open and receptive to technical solutions	People often resist acknowledging adaptive challenges and potential solutions
Solutions can typically be implemented quickly, are widely accepted and do not challenge deeply held beliefs	Solutions can take a long time to implement and require experimentation, an openmind, and often changes in values, roles and relationships

That is not to say that technical problems are trivial or unimportant. It's a critical job to take care of the technical problems in our lives. But the ways we approach and solve technical and adaptive problems are remarkably different, making our ability to identify and distinguish between the two invaluable. And, as we're sure you've experienced, problems and challenges don't necessarily come as an either/or. Often, they include a combination of technical and adaptive challenges that are intertwined. In addition to differentiating between technical problems and adaptive challenges, another important distinction to explore is the difference between leadership and authority.

What's the Difference Between Leadership and Authority?

When talking about leadership, it's also quite important to distinguish the difference between leadership and authority. People often talk about leadership and authority interchangeably. In our framework, exercising leadership has little to do with what position you hold or your level of formal authority.

Authority can be defined as a bargain or exchange by which power is conferred in return for a service.[37] For example, by living in the United States, citizens confer on the police the power to write tickets, make arrests, and enforce laws in exchange for keeping order and offering protection. The work of authority includes things like protection, direction, order, and control, which is undoubtedly important work.

People in positions of authority may or may not have strong leadership skills. You can have authority without leadership, and you can certainly have leadership outside of authority. That means you can practice leadership from any position, regardless of your level of authority. Leadership is something that anyone can practice. For example, on a soccer team, the formal positions of authority are often the coaches and captain. But you don't need to be the coach or the captain to practice leadership; any player from any position has the ability to do that.

So, why is this important context? It's important because when you're dealing with a technical problem, the solution is often provided by an authority or expert in the field. When dealing with an adaptive challenge, there is no clear-cut answer and there isn't always an authority to turn to. It's up to all of us, in the family, group, or team, to engage in the work of leadership.

Nature Unplugged Through an Adaptive Leadership Lens

The question then becomes, is overconnection to technology and disconnection from nature a technical problem or an adaptive challenge? The answer we've come to is that it's both, and it's equally important to address both. The technical problems are solved by experts and authorities in the field with tips, tricks, and tools to create better boundaries with technology and reconnect with nature. Some examples of these "hacks" are finding a home for your phone, creating a technology-free zone in your house, and scheduling time in your calendar for work or study breaks to go outside and experience nature unplugged.

The adaptive piece is more difficult to pinpoint and address concisely. It's creating a shift in your lifestyle and reevaluating your values and priorities as an individual, as a family, or as a team. The solutions to the adaptive challenges don't just come from the experts in the field. Leadership from all levels (parents, kids, teachers, coworkers, managers, etc.) is required. One of the reasons adaptive challenges are difficult to face and address is that they require us to give up things we are familiar with, find comfort in, or love.

In *The Practice of Adaptive Leadership*, Heifetz and Linsky write, "Systems, organizations, families, and communities resist dealing with adaptive challenges because doing so requires changes that partly involve an experience of loss."[38] On the one hand, it can be easy to become discouraged when realizing change requires loss; but on the other hand, it can be quite empowering. The truth is that all changes require loss of some sort. Think about any change or adaptation you've gone through—going on a diet or starting a new exercise routine, dealing with a health challenge, starting or ending a relationship. There is going to be some level of loss and disappointment in any of those. If we're not prepared to deal with the disappointment that loss brings, or if we try to avoid or deny the loss, the change will either never happen or will be unsuccessful. This must be faced and understood from the start.

To date, much of the work in this field has been rooted in technical solutions to correct technology overuse and inspire a reconnection to nature. Our aim is to take a more holistic approach by addressing both the technical and adaptive aspects of this issue. In the chapters ahead we'll share our favorite and most effective technical solutions first. It's critical to get the technical pieces in order right away. Then, we'll step into the deeper, adaptive work. We will offer questions to inspire conversation and reflection, as well as provide resources to help you tackle the challenges of living in the digital age as an individual, family, a team, or as part of a larger community. We approach the work here the same way we do with our coaching clients. We do not solve our clients' problems for them. Instead, we help them get out of their own way, offer resources and tools, and empower them to find solutions from within.

Understanding Your Values and What's Important to You

Let's return to the concept of time. Both knowing that our time is precious and embracing that time is finite can be strong motivators for living life with intention. Part of the process of stepping into leadership, becoming more intentional, and increasing our self-awareness is getting in touch with our values. Connecting with our values helps us understand what's important to us and prompts us to explore what we really want. From there, we can begin to examine our behaviors and actions to see if they are in alignment with our values.

So, what are values? Simply put, values are deeply held beliefs that are important to us. They inform what we think is good or bad, desirable or undesirable, and what we like or dislike. When we are in touch with our core values, we can use them to guide our behaviors—including the way we use technology, and how we connect to nature, ourselves, and each other. Knowing our values is like having a compass or GPS while hiking in an unfamiliar place. If we know where true north is, it's much easier to find our path. Surprisingly, many of us aren't fully aware or conscious of what our core values are.

Knowing our values helps us stay in touch with what we want, or don't want, when it comes to technology. It's much easier to navigate the digital age with our values fresh in our minds. If we don't know what our values are or if we lose sight of them, it's easy to get lost or distracted by all the noise that the attention economy creates. The following exercise is a starting point to step into our values. We will dive into this more deeply in Chapter 9 when we focus on our inner alignment.

Activity: Core Values Sort

What do you value? Use this activity as an opportunity to discover and understand what you value most in life. Follow the steps below, completing one at a time (don't skip ahead!).

Acceptance	Curiosity	Humor	Performance	Stability
Accountability	Daring	Inclusiveness	Personal Growth	Success
Achievement	Decisiveness	Independence	Playfulness	Teamwork
Advancement	Dependability	Individuality	Popularity	Thankfulness
Adventure	Diversity	Innovation	Power	Thoughtfulness
Advocacy	Empathy	Intelligence	Preparedness	Traditionalism
Ambition	Enthusiasm	Intuition	Proactivity	Trustworthiness
Appreciation	Ethics	Joy	Professionalism	Understanding
Balance	Excellence	Kindness	Quality	Usefulness
Beauty	Fairness	Knowledge	Recognition	Versatility
Boldness	Family	Leadership	Relationships	Vision
Calmness	Flexibility	Learning	Resilience	Warmth
Caring	Freedom	Love	Resourcefulness	Wealth
Challenge	Friendship	Loyalty	Risk Taking	Well-Being
Cheerfulness	Fun	Mindfulness	Safety	Wisdom
Collaboration	Generosity	Motivation	Security	Zeal
Commitment	Grace	Open-Mindedness	Self-Control	_____
Community	Happiness	Optimism	Selflessness	_____
Cooperation	Health	Passion	Service	_____
Creativity	Honesty	Peace	Simplicity	_____
Credibility	Humility	Perfection	Spirituality	_____

STEP 1: Review the list of values and draw an "X" next to any that resonate with you.

STEP 2: Now underline the 15 values that feel most important to you.

STEP 3: Carefully consider the 15 values you underlined and circle your top 5.

MY CORE VALUES

After completing the core values sort, write your top five values below. Take some time to reflect on what you've chosen. Our values become our north star, guiding our behavior and attitude as we walk through life. When you are aware of your values, you can make decisions that align with them.

1. _____

2. _____

3. _____

4. _____

5. _____

PAUSE AND REFLECT

- *Was the process of choosing your core values easy and straightforward or did you find it challenging? Why might that be?*
- *How do your values affect how you act? Do they impact the way you use technology or how you connect to nature?*

PART TWO

RESET

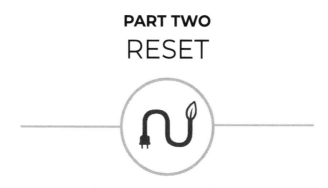

How to Create a New Relationship with Technology and Nature

While it's important to understand the problem we're facing, this book is really about stepping into the solutions. We like to think of pushing a big red reset button here. This is all about becoming more intentional with our tech and bringing more nature into our lives. We'll introduce our "Four Steps to Reset" process, which helps redefine our relationship with tech and nature. By using boundaries to minimize our daily digital distractions, we open up space in our day to include more time in nature unplugged. Nature is one of the greatest antidotes to technology overuse. In a high-tech world, we need higher doses of nature time to restore the balance. By the end of Part II, we'll emerge from our media haze and be able to focus on what's important.

CHAPTER 3

Wellness with Technology

ꞏ∿ꞏ

Technology is a useful servant,
but a dangerous master.
—Christian Lous Lange

As we've mentioned, you don't need to bury yourself in the research to understand the challenges of living in the digital age. We welcome you to continue exploring the literature if it interests you, but for our purposes we'd like to shift our focus to the path forward. As a quick reminder, we'll be looking at this challenge through the lens of adaptive leadership. It will serve as the foundation for our journey together and it will be important to remember that the challenges of living well in the digital age have both technical and adaptive components.

Both the technical and adaptive aspects of wellness with technology are equally important. So, which do you start with? In our work with clients, we've found that taking care of the technical side first tends to be most effective. The best way to step into this work is by creating boundaries with technology and reconnecting with nature. This is what we call the "Reset" phase. Tending to this important technical work creates the space for and encourages the adaptive work that will follow. In this chapter we will dive into the technical solutions that can help us live well with all of the gadgets, devices, and screens in our lives. This includes our *Four Steps to Reset* process to improve your relationship with tech and reclaim your free time.

What Does a Healthy Relationship with Technology Look Like?

This is a question we ask clients upfront and one we come back to time after time. Let's clarify that we are talking about smart devices like smartphones, tablets, computers, smart televisions, and wearable technology with web-enabled tools that connect us to a variety of digital media, software, and apps. We are not talking about your relationship with your washing machine, toaster, and vacuum—though it does seem like we're trending toward everything becoming a smart device. So, depending on when you're reading this, you may have a smart fridge that lets you know when you're low on milk and pushes an advertisement your way at the same time. What's the problem with smart devices? There's no problem with them as long as we see them for what they are. They can be fun, awesome, powerful tools that help us do some great things. But now we know they are not neutral. Specifically, the people and algorithms behind the device design, apps, and digital media we consume have an agenda: to get our attention quickly, keep it longer, and keep us coming back more often.

What does having a good relationship with technology mean, then? Think of this the same way you think about having a relationship with another person or anything else—a friend, partner, pet, or something like exercise, food, alcohol, or shopping.

- What's the quality of that relationship like?
- Is it a giving relationship? In what ways?
- Do you feel dependent on this relationship? If so, how?
- When do you typically turn to technology and your devices?
- How do you feel when you're using your smart devices?
- How do you feel after using them? Does it leave you feeling fulfilled and content or frustrated and lonely? Or both?

Remember, there's no right or wrong answer when it comes to your relationship with technology. We are simply gathering data points, not pointing fingers.

When you pause to think about this, you probably have a good sense of what your relationship with technology is like. The fact that you are reading this book shows that you're aware of this relationship and you are seeking to improve it. You've done some reflective work and are already in touch with what aspects of tech you appreciate most and what aspects seem to get in the way. That's the information you'll need to find the solutions that fit you best.

Now the question shifts to, what do YOU want out of your relationship with technology? That's the million-dollar question, and one we don't typically ask ourselves. This is a missed opportunity. Once we know what we want, we can create a clear intention and set parameters and boundaries that help us stay in alignment. When working with our clients, a big part of the work upfront is helping them see more clearly where the benefits are and where the distractions are, and distinguishing between the two. Then, we support them in creating a plan to become the driver in their relationship with technology instead of sitting in the back seat. This will be one of our main objectives in this chapter.

Using Boundaries to Find Balance

Our passion and deeper interest lives in the solutions, not the problem. Finding balance and wellness with the technology in our lives is the exciting part. Until we start changing our behaviors and taking actionable steps, we're really just swimming circles around the problem. The ability to create and maintain boundaries is critical to developing a healthy relationship with the tech and media in your life.

You may already be familiar with the term "boundaries," as it's become quite popular in recent years. Whether in the realm of psychology, relationships and dating, or health and wellness, you can find a lot of "how-to" information for creating and maintaining boundaries. The way we talk about boundaries here may be different from what you've heard elsewhere. We like to think of boundaries as creating a container. That container holds and protects the things you want and keeps out the things you don't. With boundaries, we're focusing on the management of three things: time, task, and territory. Let's take a closer look at these.

TIME	**TASK**	**TERRITORY**
Managing the amount of time dedicated to tasks and activities by setting time limits or ranges.	Specific, intentional focus on one singular task (no multitasking!).	Creating and protecting the space that you're in by minimizing distractions and setting ideal conditions.

When we hold and attend to these three boundaries consciously throughout the day we feel happier, healthier, and more satisfied. We get more done and, if you can believe it, have more free time.

Sonya's Story: Boundaries in Action

The final requirement when I was in graduate school at the University of San Diego was a thesis paper. It was a big task, with the end product hovering around fifty pages. The work was front-loaded, meaning the bulk of the work had to be done before even starting to write the final paper. I was working full-time and going to school full-time. The project often felt overwhelming, and I continued to put it off and avoid it whenever it popped into my mind. Finally I reached a tipping point where not working on it became more stressful than working on it. To reduce anxiety, I started to break the project down into manageable chunks and create internal deadlines. Allocating windows of **time** for the work helped with accountability, and I committed to 5:00–7:00 p.m. on Thursday and Friday evenings and 8:00–11:00 a.m. on Saturdays.

Half the battle was deciding to commit to working on the project (the **task**). Once that was settled and the days and time blocks were set, I put them on the calendar and made sure I wouldn't have any other competing priorities to distract me. After a week or two of solid work on the final project, I started to become more aware and intentional about where I was working, or the **territory.** Sometimes I worked at home, but that was often challenging because I felt pulled or tempted to do a lot of other things besides work on this project. When working from home was the most practical option, I cleared space at the dining room table, put away the phone, and minimized background noise like TV or music. Occasionally I even turned the Wi-Fi off so I wouldn't be tempted to browse social media, check email, or look at the news. There was a lot of trial and error, but eventually I found a rhythm and managed my boundaries effectively. I'm happy to share that the project was completed on time, and it actually became part of the inspiration for this book.

~

While it's easier said than done, without the conscious management of these three boundaries, our chances for success plummet. That's not to say that once you have these things set that other distractions or unforeseen circumstances won't come up. They probably will. But, you'll be much more prepared to respond and adjust, having thought about time, task, and territory beforehand.

So, how does this relate to finding a solution to tech and screen-time overload? Think about creating and holding boundaries as foundational for being intentional with tech. Boundaries are tools that help us use technology in ways that serve us well. Without boundaries, we are at the whim of whatever is happening around us and lose touch with how we really want to be using our time. Without boundaries, completing the thesis is less likely to happen. Without boundaries, we're more likely to be distracted and miss something important a friend, colleague, partner, or family member tells us. In terms of tech use and screen time, when we don't have boundaries, we spend our time the way tech programmers and developers prompt and encourage us to: We get sucked into the vortex of the attention economy, where time and intention begin to slip away from us.

Now, it is possible to create too many boundaries, where every second of our day is assigned a specific task. That's not the goal either. While having no boundaries can be a recipe for disaster, so too can being overly bound. It's important to allow for free time and fun during your day, to find a balance between doing and being. When we talk about the practice of holding and managing boundaries skillfully, it's really about the ability to loosen or tighten boundaries depending on that particular situation. For example, how you manage your boundaries at a work meeting is different from how you manage your boundaries having a casual dinner with friends.

Using boundaries is a critical piece in cultivating wellness in the digital age. Remember, time is finite. When we choose to spend our time on one thing, we're simultaneously choosing not to spend our time on other things. Setting boundaries helps create space in our day and lives for the things we want, enjoy, and appreciate. Once we have the boundaries working and in place, we can intentionally fill that space with what brings us joy, connection, and aliveness.

Digital vs. Analog

In addition to boundary work, we're also always on the lookout for how to bring more analog experiences into our lives. In a 2017 *New York Times* article, "Our Love Affair with Technology is Over," author David Sax digs into why there has been an increase in popularity of analog items like old-fashioned print books, journals, and vinyl records.[39] Sax makes a great case for seeking balance between digital and analog. While tech and screens and apps will continue to have their place, it's useful to explore where we can slow down, breathe, and do things the old-fashioned way.

Why would you use analog items when there's probably "an app for that"? As Sax describes, going analog is a wonderful way to find balance and take a break from the digital world. In our personal lives and in working with clients, we've found that incorporating more analog activities can be a wonderful solution to feeling overwhelmed by all things digital.

Let's take a closer look at what we mean by digital and analog. The technical definition of analog is data transmitted through a continuous stream. The definition of digital is data transmitted through ones and zeroes. But really, the way we are talking about these terms is a little different. Analog refers to things that are old school, authentic, low or no-tech and nostalgic. Things like board games, printed books, and vinyl records. Digital refers to things that are high tech and smart tech. For example, video games, apps, games on your phone, e-books, etc.

Many of us have developed a romanticized relationship with all things digital. With this comes a mindset that digital makes everything better and easier. And, as we know, there is some truth to that, but it's not the whole truth. Going digital with everything isn't all that it's chalked up to be.

As Sax describes in the article, there's been a resurgence in popularity of analog items. Like a pendulum, we've swung a little too far to the digital side. We seem starved for tactile experiences and are swinging slightly back toward the analog side. There is something satisfying and rich about physically moving a figure across a board game versus swiping across a screen. Similarly, there's something gratifying about reading a physical book: holding it, flipping through the pages, the scent of the paper. All of it captures our attention in a way that an e-book doesn't.

While many of us enjoy analog experiences, studies show that in some cases going analog is more effective and better for us, not simply more enjoyable. In a 2014 study published in *Psychological Science*, Pam Mueller of Princeton University and Daniel Oppenheimer of the University of California, Los Angeles, looked at the differences between how note-taking by hand and by computer affects learning.[40] The study showed that when people type their notes, they tend to do so verbatim. They write exactly what the professor or teacher says. When people take notes by hand, they are forced to be more selective in what they write because writing is slower than typing. The research suggests that this extra processing of the material helps students retain the information more effectively.

The Myth of Multitasking

I (Sebastian) was a big fan of multitasking for much of my life. I consider myself a recovering multitasker, though it's still something that's easy for me to slip back into without awareness. As Sonya will tell you, I can get pretty excited about getting things done and filling my day to the max. Getting one task done is great, but getting multiple tasks done at the same time is even better, right?! The concept sounds wonderful, but my experience of multitasking didn't usually go so well. After multitasking I would typically end up feeling frazzled, with very little to show for it in terms of results.

It turns out, I'm not alone in feeling this way when attempting to multitask. Dr. Larry Rosen, whom we introduced earlier in this book, is also an expert in multitasking. When we interviewed Dr. Rosen, he shared that most of the time that we think we're multitasking, we're not. Rosen says, "What we can multitask with are very simple tasks. For example, I can walk and chew gum at the same time without falling over my feet. But, I can't drive and be on my phone without difficulty or a slower response time. Both tasks have to be fairly automatic in order to truly multitask."

What we think is multitasking is actually task switching, because we cannot focus on two things at the same time. He went on to explain what's going on in the brain when we attempt to multitask, or more accurately, task switch. "What's happening in the brain when you think you're multitasking is that your brain is allocating blood flow to a certain area, which brings glucose and oxygen to that particular area. Then, that excites the neurons and they send biochemical signals to other neurons, and you start thinking about something. Now, when you change your thought, when you task switch, the blood starts to flow away from where it was going and into a totally different area of your brain. You are now thinking of something totally different. In the meantime, what you were thinking about is no longer activated in your brain. So, it takes you a long time—some studies have shown it takes up to 25 minutes—for you to return to what you actually want to be working on."

Dr. Rosen shared an example of a study he and his colleagues did that highlights the issues with multitasking by looking at the study habits of students. Here's how the study worked. They observed middle school, high school, and college students studying at home. The observer would typically be a friend or someone well known so that the experience didn't feel intrusive or threatening. They told the students, "We want you to study something important for just fifteen minutes." They then said, "We're going to watch you studying," and the observer sat there with a clipboard and observed. Every minute the observer marked down whether the student was on task or not, and if they were on task, they noted what they were doing. The observer also marked down what websites were on their screens, and other relevant information.

What Dr. Rosen and his team found was fascinating. First, it didn't seem to make a difference what age the subjects were, whether it be middle school, high school, or college; they all stayed on task for about the same amount of time during the 15-minute observation period. Second, on average, studying was on task about 60% of the time or about 10 of the 15 minutes. This was surprising to us, considering the students knew they were being watched the entire time. What the researchers found was a consistent pattern where students studied for a few minutes and then became distracted, studied for a few more minutes and then became distracted again. Dr. Rosen noted, "What we are really looking at is an average attention span of 3–6 minutes, and this finding has been replicated in other studies. Remember then, if you have to reactivate that part of your brain, that takes time. So if you're only studying for 3–6 minutes and then you get distracted, even just for a minute or two, you don't just go back to exactly where you left off studying before. It takes time to get back on track." He continued, "We have found these numbers consistent across the board, and the takeaway is that task switching simply is not a good strategy. Yes, you can eventually do as good a job of studying as someone who's not interrupted, but it takes you much longer and you end up with much higher stress levels."

In our work, we've noticed this isn't unique to young people. Research shows that it impacts adults just as much as it impacts grade school and college students. It's not an age thing, it's a human thing. As Dr. Rosen likes to put it, "It turns out that this is unique to our human brains."

Yes, yes, we know. Task switching and distraction both predate smartphones. However, there is plenty of evidence that our smartphones and other devices are making things much worse. This is due to a variety of things like notifications, brightly colored icons, and all of the factors that contribute to the attention economy. How then do we resist the pull to multitask? Boundaries! Using boundaries is a great way to minimize or avoid task switching, and here are some of our favorite strategies for putting boudaries into action.

Four Steps to Reset Your Relationship with Tech

When it comes to boundary work and resetting your relationship with technology, it's helpful to have clear steps and guidance to get started. Otherwise, it can be tricky to figure out what to do first. We've developed a four-step process to help jump-start this reset. This was inspired by our research, working with clients, and experience in our own relationship navigating the pulls of technology. We recommend starting with these steps as a foundation. While the four steps are simple, they are enough to completely change your relationship with tech. And, you can certainly go deeper if you're interested in doing so by exploring the additional tips included at the end of this chapter.

Step 1: Create a Digital Curfew
Step 2: No Tech in the Bedroom
Step 3: Find a Home for Your Phone
Step 4: Schedule Unplugged Time

STEP 1: CREATE A DIGITAL CURFEW

Your "digital curfew" is the time you'll put your devices—phone, tablet, laptop, TV, and video games—to bed for the night, and the time you'll start using them again in the morning. We'd recommend 1–2 hours before you go to sleep and after you wake up. For example, you might turn off and put away your devices at 8:00 p.m. every night and not use them again until 8:00 a.m. the next day. At the very least, try to make a habit of brushing your teeth before checking your phone in the morning.

STEP 2: NO TECH IN THE BEDROOM

This may sound radical if you've currently got a lot of technology in your bedroom, but this is a game changer. The main issue is that devices in the bedroom tend to stimulate you, either with bright light, sound, or engaging content. None of those are great for preserving your ability to get a good night's sleep. If your main hang-up is that you use your phone as your alarm, remember that analog alarm clocks still exist!

STEP 3: FIND A HOME FOR YOUR PHONE

Create a place where your phone lives when you're not intentionally using it. This could be a charging station in your living room or a basket in your entryway. Right when you get home, it's where your phone goes, and it stays there until you're ready to intentionally use it again. Otherwise, you may end up wandering all over the house with your phone in your pocket or attached to your hand!

STEP 4: SCHEDULE UNPLUGGED TIME

Now that we have created some great boundaries, this step helps to create space for unplugged time. We recommend scheduling at least 60 minutes per day of unplugged time into your calendar (outside of your digital curfew time). If you have the opportunity to get out into nature unplugged, it's ideal but not necessary. The focus here is on creating breaks in our tech and screen time throughout the day. This unplugged time could be all at once during an unplugged walk, workout, or perhaps analog craft or reading time. Or, you can break it down into smaller chunks if that works better for your schedule. One of our favorite ways to get in our unplugged time is by taking short unplugged breaks from work. It's so easy to get in the habit of going from working on screens to taking work breaks by checking the news or social media on screens. Taking intentional unplugged breaks, whether it's a quick walk or stretch, can be such a great way to give our brains a break in order to recharge.

More Tech Tips

If you want a quick and effective reset for your relationship with technology, we recommend starting with the four steps above. If you're looking to go deeper, the following section has a few more of our favorite tips for getting your tech boundaries in order.

"BOOKENDING" YOUR DAY

This goes along with setting a digital curfew. We highly recommend bookending your day with a tech-free morning routine and a tech-free evening routine. This could include things like stretching, meditation, prayer, tech-free exercise, reading a physical book, or doing a crossword puzzle. Find what works for you and explore working it into your schedule. Bookending your day is a wonderful way to create positive structure in your life, and it does wonders to help protect and enhance the quality of your sleep.

CREATE TECH-FREE SPACES

This one is pretty intuitive. You're creating a space in your house that is tech-free. That space can be an entire room, a specific corner of a room, or a table or sitting area within a room. What's helpful here is normalizing tech-free spaces in your home. It's a way to create some etiquette around technology in your household and manage expectations of each other. Examples of this are no tech in the bedroom, tech-free dinner tables, and tech-free play or activity rooms.

CREATE TECH-SPECIFIC SPACES

Creating tech-specific spaces is helpful too. Designating spaces that are meant to use technology creates a clear purpose and function of the devices in those spaces. It also helps create expectations that technology wouldn't be used outside of those spaces. Good examples here are computer stations, offices, and entertainment rooms. This is also connected to finding a home for your phone. When you're home, the more that you can use your phone in tech-specific areas, the more intentional your phone use will become. This also works well for other devices. If you work from home, consider putting your laptop in a drawer or leaving it in your office when done with work for the day.

CREATE WINDOWS OF TIME FOR COMMUNICATION

Just because we can call, text, and email friends, family, and colleagues 24/7 doesn't mean it's a good practice. As much as possible, set specific times to call, text, and email. This is important for time management and productivity. It's also hugely helpful for staying present in the office, classroom, or when you're with family and friends. An example of this would be to only look at emails from 9–10 a.m., 1–2 p.m., and 4–5 p.m. Maybe you only text a few times a day: once in the morning, once at midday, and once in the evening. If we're not intentional, calls, texts, messaging, and emails can easily cause interruptions and take over much (if not all!) of our day.

SET SCREEN TIME LIMITS

Almost all smartphones, tablets, and computers have settings that allow you to set screen time limits. You can set general phone usage time limits or time limits for specific apps and games. You can even use screen time limits to manage your communication windows. This is a great way to hold yourself accountable, raise your screen time awareness, and encourage intentional technology use.

GO ANALOG WHEN POSSIBLE

Going analog or low-tech is a great way to balance and create boundaries with your tech use. Ask yourself if you really need to be using technology for any given task. If you don't, if using technology creates more distraction than benefit, consider an analog alternative. By analog we mean low-tech or no-tech. For example, read a physical book instead of reading on a tablet or Kindle. When you have a chance, write your to-do list in a journal instead of on your phone or computer.

In a world that seems to be heading toward a digitally saturated future, we encourage you to take some time and reflect on what ways you can incorporate analog experiences into your life.

Here are some ideas to get you started:

- Read physical books instead of e-books.
- Arrange for a friend or family game night (with analog games) once a week or month.
- When traveling, experiment with using paper maps and atlases instead of GPS. (It's a great skill to develop, especially when there's no cell service.)
- Listen to vinyl records (or go to live music) in addition to streaming digital music.
- Create your own music.
- Take notes by hand with pen and paper instead of typing.
- Use a film camera or Polaroid instead of a digital camera or smartphone.

TURN OFF AUTOPLAY

Did you know you can turn off autoplay? YouTube and Netflix allow you to switch autoplay off in their settings menu. It can be a little tricky to do (the tech companies don't want us messing with autoplay), but is well worth the time to change. Turning off autoplay gives you back the power, and choice, to watch the next episode or not.

TURN OFF NOTIFICATIONS

Most apps on our phones, tablets, and computers push alerts and notifications to us on a consistent basis. These include banners that float over our home screens, sounds, or number icons to show how many emails or notifications are waiting for us. Decide what you need to know urgently and turn off all your other notifications. For example, we only allow call and text notifications to come through. You can manage these settings in your device's settings section, though sometimes you may need to go into a specific app to make changes. Also be sure to check out the "Do Not Disturb" feature now available on most smart devices. You can set daily times (like 10:00 p.m. to 7:00 a.m.) when no alerts, notifications, calls, or texts come through, or just turn on this feature during important meetings, calls, or quality time with friends and family.

CLEAR YOUR HOME SCREEN

Clearing the home screen of our phones has been one of the most powerful tips we've put into practice. The home screen on your phone is the screen you see once you've unlocked your phone (think about this as the desktop on your computer). This is where you would typically see all of your favorite apps. The practice here is to completely clear your home screen so no apps are visible. First, create a folder that lives on the bottom dock of your phone. Once you have your folder ready, move all of your apps into that folder, leaving your home screen totally clear. Moving forward, instead of just looking through your home screen for the app you want to use, now you'll use the search feature to find the particular app you want. This forces us to be much more intentional in how we use our phone.

Activity: Four Steps to Reset (in Action)

CREATE A DIGITAL CURFEW

I will create the following digital curfew:

Each morning we will not use technology/devices before:

_____ (a.m.)

Each evening we will put our devices to sleep by:

_____ (p.m.)

NO TECH IN THE BEDROOM

I will keep the following devices out of the bedroom:
- ☐ Cell Phone
- ☐ TV
- ☐ Laptop

- ☐ Tablet
- ☐ Computer
- ☐ Video Games
- ☐ _____
- ☐ _____
- ☐ _____
- ☐ _____

FIND A HOME FOR YOUR PHONE

The home for my phone will be located:

- ☐ In a basket by the front door
- ☐ At a charging station in the living room
- ☐ _____
- ☐ _____

SCHEDULE UNPLUGGED TIME

I will unplug every day for _____ minutes. My intention is to take:

- ☐ One long break of at least 60 minutes
- ☐ Two 30-minute breaks
- ☐ A few smaller breaks of 5–15 minutes each
- ☐ _____
- ☐ _____

PAUSE AND REFLECT

- *How does technology use impact your relationship with other people and the world around you?*
- *What boundaries do you already have in place to help support a healthy relationship with technology and digital media?*
- *What would be the most meaningful and useful boundary you could start implementing right now?*

CHAPTER 4

A Natural Solution

ᘯ

*Thousands of tired, nerve-shaken, over-civilized people
are beginning to find out that going to the mountains
is going home; that wildness is a necessity;
and that mountain parks and reservations are useful
not only as fountains of timber and irrigating rivers,
but as fountains of life.*
—John Muir

Up until now, much of our focus and attention has been on tech, screens, and media. We'd like you to step into a new space now (metaphorically speaking), away from devices, Wi-Fi, and outlets, and into the fresh air and sunlight. This is a space that is wild and full of possibilities, a space that is refreshing and rejuvenating, like walking through a mountain meadow on a cool spring morning. This is the second part of the reset phase. Now that we've created more space and time in our day by resetting our relationship with technology, it's time to focus our energy on bringing more nature into our lives.

The natural world is in many ways the complete opposite of the digital world. If screens, wires, devices, and outlets are on one end of the spectrum, trees, clouds, and vast mountain ranges are on the other. And, as we will explore, many of the negative outcomes from being overconnected to tech are remedied by time spent in nature, unplugged. Again, we are not anti-tech; our focus is on finding balance.

As a reminder, our species has been inhabiting Earth for around 200,000 years (and our earlier ancestors are estimated to have been around between five and seven million years ago). Civilization as we've come to know it only began around 6,000 years ago, the industrialization started in the 1800s, and the digital revolution began in the

1980s. From an evolutionary perspective, we've been living amongst the fields, forests, and mountains for the majority of our existence. It's only very recently that we've moved to a modern, high-tech lifestyle that is relatively disconnected from the natural world.

Connection with nature is our birthright. It's also foundational for wellness in the digital age. As we've already mentioned, research on the benefits of nature has been mounting in recent years. We'll offer an overview of the benefits of nature, why nature is a perfect antidote to screen time, nature doses, and our favorite tips, recommendations, and ideas for bringing more nature into your life.

What Does a Healthy Relationship with Nature Look Like?

When we ask people what a healthy relationship with *technology* looks like, responses flood in. When we ask folks what a healthy relationship with *nature* looks like, responses tend to trickle in. Perhaps it's useful to clarify what we mean by nature, as the term can feel a bit abstract. What do we mean when we talk about nature? We aren't necessarily talking about pristine wilderness or untouched ecosystems. While those are wonderful to experience, they can be quite challenging to access. Rather, we are using the term in a broader sense. When we talk about nature, we are referring to any aspect of the physical world, including plants, animals, landscapes, or other natural features as opposed to man-made creations.

When we first started Nature Unplugged, our vision was to provide unique outdoor experiences to individuals and families through retreats and guided nature adventures. This ranged from weekend camping trips in the local mountains of Southern California to weeklong nature and surfing retreats in Central America and abroad. That work is important, and there are huge benefits that come from taking extended trips (even a few days) into nature. However, we realized early on that this model wasn't complete. What we noticed after facilitating retreats, and even attending retreats ourselves, was that you can have awesome retreat experiences but you'll often go back to the way things were post-retreat without much lasting change. Instead of providing intensive nature experiences, we became much more interested in helping others discover ways to bring nature into their lives on a daily basis.

To use an analogy around diet and nutrition, we came to see the retreat model as similar to eating poorly day to day and then going on a three-day juice cleanse. Of course, the juice cleanse is hugely helpful, but it doesn't necessarily address the day-to-day lifestyle and eating patterns. It's more important to focus on getting the proper nutrition every day. Then, the occasional juice cleanse is a wonderful boost to your clean eating lifestyle, but it's not necessary. It works the same with nature connection. The more meaningful work is examining your lifestyle and addressing your daily connection with nature. Then, much like the juice cleanse, a retreat or camping trip will enhance and build on your relationship with nature. This focus on day-to-day lifestyle quickly became our passion and in turn became the foundation of our work.

If connection to nature isn't just about frolicking in untouched wilderness, what does it look like in our daily lives? Here are some possibilities:

- Gardening
- Lying under a tree
- Playing in the grass in your backyard
- Backpacking through a national park
- Walking through an urban park or green space
- Watching the clouds through a kitchen window
- Stargazing
- Interacting with a pet
- Birding
- Outdoor exercise
- Ocean and outdoor water sports

As you can see, it doesn't require much to connect with nature. Certainly, not all nature is created equal. The benefits and exposure to nature when backpacking in the mountains of Patagonia is going to be different from walking through a small urban green space. However, the point is that you don't have to go halfway across the world to find a deep connection with nature and can experience the benefits without needing too much time or resources. Connecting with nature and bringing nature into our lives on a daily basis can be simple and quick.

What does a healthy relationship with nature look like to you? Does this question feel different to you now? What comes to mind? Perhaps it's spending regular time at a local park or green space. Maybe it brings up thoughts and images of having more plants around, or hanging pictures of beautiful landscapes in your home. For some, it may spark thoughts of environmental justice or environmental stewardship.

Different people have different ways of connecting with nature and varying amounts of time and resources to do so. Similar to our relationship with tech, the purpose is to explore this relationship and gather data points. We are working to expand our awareness and our understanding of how we relate and connect with nature. And, that we are intentional about developing and nourishing that relationship. As we have learned by now, if we aren't intentional about cultivating our relationship with nature, and if we aren't intentional about our boundaries with tech, our time and attention will get swept away by our screens and devices and we'll fall into the vortex that is the attention economy.

When working with our clients to create healthier relationships with nature, our aim is to explore what works best for that individual, family, or team. Our intention here is to do the same for you. By the time you finish this chapter, our goal is for you to have the resources and tools to elevate your relationship with nature and find ways to incorporate more of it into your life.

Looking Back at Nature

A wonderful way to begin exploring this topic is by reflecting on how your relationship with nature began. Where in nature did you play as a kid and how did that inspire you? Or, if you're a youngster, where in nature do you play and how does that inspire you? Pause here for a moment and reflect on your childhood connection with nature. Remember, your nature place doesn't have to be anything too remote or exotic. It can be as simple as playing catch in your grandparents' backyard or climbing a tree in your neighborhood. Whatever place comes to mind is perfect.

Most of us have some sort of memory of playing in nature as children. This reflection can serve as a wonderful reminder and can provide the foundation for continuing to build up your relationship with nature. We were both fortunate enough to have had places to play in nature when we were growing up: from exploring the hills and fields of Valley Forge National Historical Park outside of Philadelphia to swimming and diving through the waves in Southern California. It's incredible when we reflect back on those times and realize how influential they were and continue to be for us.

Sonya's Story: The Wild Forest

It was a 10-to-15-minute walk from my house in a suburb outside of Philadelphia to the edge of Valley Forge National Historical Park. Everything seems larger when you're young, but the park always felt enormous to me. Different seasons would bring different reasons to visit the park. The summer would bring opportunities for picnics and barbeques with friends and family. The spring and fall offered changing leaves and cooler weather, perfect for long walks. The winter brought snow and abundant hillsides to sled down (some popular and crowded and a few secret and hidden). As a kid, I was less fascinated by the historical context of the park and more impressed by the grand wilderness on the edge of my suburban life.

There's one particular memory I have of the park when I was sixteen years old that seemed rather insignificant at the time, but now seems pivotal to a shift in my relationship with nature. The park features many roads, walking paths, and trails used to explore the historical sites and move easily from one point to another. I tended to stick to those designated travel paths without feeling compelled to step off them. That is, until I was spending some time in the park with my friend Josh, and he simply stepped off the trail and set off in a different direction. He started heading up a slight incline into a more heavily wooded area, looked back and said, "Let's go this way." It made me slightly uncomfortable, but I shrugged it off and followed, curious if he knew where he was going.

We walked deeper into the woods for a while, and I started to notice how different the ground felt beneath my feet: cushy, almost, with all the fallen leaves and tinder in each step. It felt quiet and still and full of life all at the same time. Josh stopped ahead of me and I naturally slowed behind him, coming to a stop just beside him. As I was about to ask him why we'd stopped, I heard a rustling of leaves and movement a few feet ahead of us and to the right. About ten feet from where we were standing was a beautiful deer. For a moment it froze, looking at us without turning its head, and then quickly went on its way, nibbling at the brush as it went around us. We stood silently, for maybe five minutes, standing together and watching the deer move along.

Before that experience, deer were not particularly interesting to me. Living so close to the park, and with wooded and natural areas spotted throughout our community, I saw deer daily. Actually, deer had a reputation for being a nuisance where I grew up because they would come right up to the local houses and eat all of the plants and flowers. That, or they were known as driving hazards, often being hit by cars near dusk and dawn. That's what deer were to me, before that moment with Josh in the park. Then all of a sudden, in just a few minutes, deer became beautiful, mysterious animals that I got to live beside. That deer was doing exactly as I was, quietly wandering through the woods. I felt incredibly aware of myself, my surroundings, and connected to Josh, the deer, and the forest. I felt wild and peaceful, and there was nowhere I'd rather have been.

That moment helped to shift my perspective and experience of nature. It was a reminder that the trees, rolling hills, rivers, and oceans were more than pretty scenery. It brought me back in touch with a childlike wonder that had been fading away as I got older. I started to see nature the way I had as a child—a wild place full of possibilities where animals roamed, insects burrowed in the ground, and birds nested. It was beauty and adventure rolled up together. Being more attentive and curious radically changed how I experienced nature. It's twenty years later, and I still think about that moment a lot. Ultimately, it's what pointed me in this direction. Since then, I've been trying to create space for others to have experiences in nature like the one I had. To encourage more time outside, unplugged and engaged.

Sebastian's Story: At Home in the Ocean

When I think back on where in nature I played as a kid, there is one place that comes to mind: the beach (and ocean). As I mentioned at the beginning of the book, I was fortunate to grow up on the coast of Southern California in the beautiful town of La Jolla. Both my parents were avid beachgoers, and many of my earliest memories are of mixing it up on the sand and in the water. From early on, the beach became a cornerstone of my life. It was a magical place full of wonder and somewhere that I could be wild and free. I could spend hours (and often did) swimming and playing in the waves and exploring the beach.

Some of my earliest memories of playing in the ocean were with my dad at the La Jolla Cove, our favorite local beach. An amazing aspect of the Cove is that, because of its sheltered waters, it's teeming with sea life. My dad would swim me out into the deeper waters, and along the way we would greet all sorts of marine life, including a variety of fish, my favorite being the bright orange Garibaldi. We'd also come across seals and sea lions, and the occasional moray eel. The more time I spent at the Cove (and in the ocean), the more it became like a second home to me. I came to know it inside and out. Spending time at the Cove was like being in a wonderland. When I wasn't swimming or snorkeling, there were tide pools and caves to explore, or I'd play games with my dad on the sand.

After my dad died and we spread his ashes in the ocean, my connection with the ocean (and nature) deepened greatly. It was not only my favorite place to play; it became much more than that. The ocean became a refuge for me and a place to go where I felt close to my dad. Even though he wasn't physically there, I felt like his spirit was in the water, sand, seaweed, and every aspect of that environment. That combination of play, fun, and freedom along with something deeper and sacred really fueled my connection with nature.

My early memories of playing at the Cove have inspired and influenced my life greatly. And, it has served as a foundation for me to continue to deepen my connection with nature. While I enjoyed all sorts of ocean activities, like swimming, bodysurfing, bodyboarding (boogieboarding), and surfing, my very favorite was bodyboarding. As I got older, I became obsessed with the sport and spent as much time as I could in the waves honing my skills. My passion for bodyboarding eventually led to a career as a professional bodyboarder. Through bodyboarding, I had the opportunity to travel the world, exploring and experiencing some of the best waves around.

During my time traveling, an interesting shift took place. Initially with my travels and career bodyboarding, my sole focus was on getting the best waves I possibly could. It was all about performance. As

I continued to travel, I found myself more drawn to learn about the geography, culture, and natural history of the places I had the opportunity to visit. I began to research and study geography and the natural world. Prior to this, my focus had been so intensely on bodyboarding that school and my studies through much of middle school and high school took a backseat. I initially chose not to go to college because of my pursuit of bodyboarding. As I traveled and this spark for learning grew inside me, I decided to go back and pursue a BA in Geography and Environmental Policy.

Since then, much of my career and focus both personally and professionally have had to do with connection to nature. When I reflect back on my journey, it's amazing to see how much of it stemmed from my early days of passion and play in the ocean. I'm not sure where I would be without it. Of course, not everyone's path is directly connected to their early days of play in nature, but I would wager that it plays a bigger role than many people think. Taking the time to look back and reflect is a wonderful way to make those connections.

Indoor Creatures

While it's helpful to reflect on our early experience with nature, it's also important to step into the present and examine our relationship with nature now. How does your relationship with nature today compare to when you were a kid? For many of us, those early days of play and adventure have faded into the background—which makes sense. With adulthood comes more responsibilities, less free time, conflicting priorities, and so forth. Comparing our relationship with nature over time, from when we were kids to now, helps us see and understand what's changed and what has prompted those changes.

Sonya's Story: 9 to 5

I didn't fully realize how much of an indoor creature I had become until a few years into my last nine-to-five job at a local university. I asked my partner Sebastian one night over dinner how his day was and what he had done. He worked in the wellness and outdoor industry and had a flexible and variable schedule. He shared that he had an outdoor coaching session, taught an open-air yoga class, went for a surf break, and then did some emails and computer work in the afternoon. I smiled and reflected on my day, where I stayed inside the same building the entire day, either in my office or a meeting room.

We started to joke that we should choose a random weekday and strap GoPros to our heads for the entire day. We'd end up with two very different time-lapse videos. It was funny to imagine, his day full of adventure and outdoor time sprinkled with some traditional admin work compared to my desk job. And then as it sank in, it didn't feel so funny anymore. I lived a mostly sedentary, indoor life. Monday through Friday my commute to and from work took about two hours, and I worked inside an office building for about nine hours. So on a typical day I spent 11 of 16 waking hours either in traffic or sitting in an office (mostly in front of a computer screen). Yikes! How was this normal? Surely it couldn't be good for me, or anyone for that matter. But somehow it was an incredibly normal experience and existence.

This was one of my biggest inspirations for co-founding Nature Unplugged and the primary motivator for me to change my career path and lifestyle. Much of my passion for Nature Unplugged comes from a deep knowledge of what it's like to be an indoor creature and how important it was to find my way back outside. And you don't have to quit your job to find balance and reconnect to nature. My aim is to help others notice their indoor lifestyle, encourage reflection, and inspire thoughtful ways to infuse more nature into their lives in a way that works for them, their work, and their families.

Getting Outside

While it may look different from person to person, folks generally agree that time in nature is a good thing. Despite this understanding, there's a dissonance between the knowing and doing. An interesting exploration of this gap came from a 2019 Outdoor Participation Report by Outdoor Foundation.[41] The report found that about half of the U.S. population participated in outdoor recreation—including hunting, hiking, camping, fishing, or canoeing, among many more outdoor activities—at least once in 2018. Which means that just under half the population didn't participate in outdoor recreation at all in 2018. Not only are we recreating in nature less, we're going outside less. According to a 2001 study published in the *Journal of Exposure Science & Environmental Epidemiology*, the average

American spends 93% of his or her time indoors.[42]

These survey results speak to a larger trend taking place across the globe: a trend away from the countryside and into cities. According to the United Nations, we've entered the urban century, and two-thirds of our population is projected to be living in cities by 2050. Of course, there is nothing inherently wrong with this trend. It simply means we need to be more intentional about getting our nature doses. What used to happen more automatically for previous generations, who lived closer and more connected to the natural world, now needs to be sought out.

To lessen the gap between knowing and doing, inspiration and motivation often comes from understanding the benefits nature can offer. Then, it's just a matter of exploring and finding ways to bring more nature into your life on a daily basis.

Nature: The Perfect Antidote

As we studied the impact of increased screen time and the benefits of nature, it became clear that the two were intertwined. Our personal experience, our work, and the literature show that nature is the perfect antidote or counterbalance to increased screen time and high-tech life. Many of the issues and problems that tech overuse cause are directly mitigated through nature exposure. The more screen time we have in our lives, the more nature time we need to incorporate to balance it out and stay healthy.

Through research, we know that increased tech use and screen time contributes to higher instances of attention disorders and our ability to focus. The research also shows how exposure to nature can actually restore our attention and focus, offsetting the impact of screen time and tech use. Let's look more closely at this.

One of the key aspects of the psychological process of how nature can help increase one's capacity for focus is called attention restoration theory (ART).[43] Attention restoration theory proposes that spending time in nature is not only enjoyable but can also help us improve our focus and ability to concentrate.[44] One study showed that everyday exposure to green space like neighborhood parks, backyards, and so on, reduced children's attention deficit symptoms on an ongoing basis. What's more, the study explained how regular exposure to green settings comes without any of the negative side effects associated with medications.[45]

Another study in the journal *Psychological Science* looked at the cognitive benefits of interacting with nature versus spending time in urban environments. The study found that nature, which is filled with intriguing stimuli, modestly grabs attention in a bottom-up fashion, allowing top-down directed attention abilities a chance to replenish. Unlike natural environments, urban environments are filled with stimulation (i.e., bright, flashing lights, loud noises, and advertisements) that captures attention dramatically and additionally requires directed attention (e.g., to avoid being hit by a car), making them less restorative. The study went on to find that walking in nature or viewing pictures of nature can improve directed-attention abilities, thus validating attention restorative theory.[46] In other words, bottom-up attention lets the brain relax and reset, making it restorative. A welcome respite from the digital age and attention economy. On the other hand, top-down attention requires executive functioning and higher-level thinking, which demands our focused attention and eventually leads to stress, fatigue, and burnout.

Those studies just scratch the surface. The research on the benefits of nature on our physical, mental, and emotional health has been around for a long time. We're not arguing that the idea that time in nature is good for us is new. What is new, though, is the recent surge over the last fifteen to twenty years in studies related to the benefits of nature—not just their quantity but their quality.

Here are a few of the benefits that nature has to offer:
- Decreases stress—lowers blood pressure, lowers cortisol levels (the stress hormone), reduces your nervous system arousal, enhances immune system function, increases self-esteem, reduces anxiety, and improves mood.[47]
- Lessens attention deficit disorders and aggression.[48]
- Reduces feelings of isolation, boosts mood, and promotes calm.[49]
- Reduces levels of depressive and anxiety symptoms.[50]
- Attention restoration theory suggests the ability to concentrate may be restored by exposure to natural environments.[51]
- "Forest bathing" is shown to increase natural killers (NK cells)

in the immune system, which fight tumors and infections.[52]

- Boosts creativity and improves cognitive functioning and creative problem solving.[53]
- Reduces physical ailments caused by sedentary lifestyles.[54]

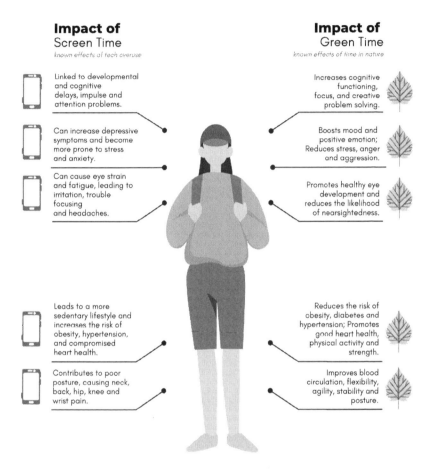

Impact of
Screen Time
known effects of tech overuse

Impact of
Green Time
known effects of time in nature

Linked to developmental and cognitive delays, impulse and attention problems.

Increases cognitive functioning, focus, and creative problem solving.

Can increase depressive symptoms and become more prone to stress and anxiety.

Boosts mood and positive emotion; Reduces stress, anger and aggression.

Can cause eye strain and fatigue, leading to irritation, trouble focusing and headaches.

Promotes healthy eye development and reduces the likelihood of nearsightedness.

Leads to a more sedentary lifestyle and increases the risk of obesity, hypertension, and compromised heart health.

Reduces the risk of obesity, diabetes and hypertension; Promotes good heart health, physical activity and strength.

Contributes to poor posture, causing neck, back, hip, knee and wrist pain.

Improves blood circulation, flexibility, agility, stability and posture.

Between the ever-growing research and our intuitive understanding that nature is critical to our well-being, especially in this digital age where technology and smart devices are everywhere, the call to action is becoming urgent. Experts across the world and across disciplines are encouraging shifts in our routines in order to bring more nature into our lives, and we agree. Now the question shifts from whether we need more nature to how much nature time we need to feel the benefits.

Nature Doses

You might think that the more time in nature, the better. And, while that's true to a certain extent, you might be surprised at how little nature time you actually need to begin feeling the benefits. It's helpful to think about this research in a medical framework, where the amount of time of nature is considered a dose. Many of the world's cultures, especially in the East, view nature as a place of healing, rejuvenation, and sustenance. It's interesting to see that Western medicine is starting to prescribe doses of nature for patients for a wide variety of reasons, including management of stress, anxiety, and depressive symptoms. With the influx of technology, more sedentary lifestyles, and rising rates of chronic diseases among children in recent decades, pediatricians are looking for alternative ways to treat their patients, including prescribing time outdoors. Here are a range of doses, both in the amount of time spent in nature and the benefits received.

FIVE MINUTES

Spending just five minutes in nature can quickly improve your mood. In a 2018 study published in *The Journal of Positive Psychology*, researchers from the University of Regina found that participants who spent five minutes sitting in nature experienced an increase in positive emotions.[55] Participants from the study were split into two groups. One group was assigned to an urban park and the other to an indoor laboratory setting. The participants were instructed to put away all of their devices and focus on their surroundings while staying seated for five minutes. Each participant was surveyed about his or her emotions and mood before and after the experiment. The results indicate that brief contact with nature reliably improved both hedonic (emotions associated with comfort and pleasure) and self-transcendent emotions (emotions associated with a higher purpose, such as compassion, gratitude, and awe).

15 MINUTES

A 15-minute walk in the woods causes measurable changes in physiology. Japanese researchers led by Yoshifumi Miyazaki at Chiba University sent 84 subjects to stroll in seven different forests, while the same number of volunteers walked around city centers. The forest walkers hit a relaxation jackpot: Overall they showed a 16 percent decrease in the stress hormone cortisol, a 2 percent drop in blood pressure, and a 4 percent drop in heart rate.[56]

90 MINUTES

Ninety minutes in nature can reduce depressive symptoms. In a 2015 study, researchers found that people who walked in natural areas, as opposed to participants who walked in high-traffic urban areas, showed decreased activity in a region of the brain associated with key factors of depression.[57] This study examined two groups: one group who walked for 90 minutes in a nature setting surrounded by oak trees and shrubs, the other along a traffic-heavy road. Before and after the walk the researchers measured participants' heart and respiration rates, and took brain scans, along with questionnaires. The researchers found the greatest changes in the brain scans, showing that neural activity in the subgenual prefrontal cortex decreased in those who walked in nature versus those who walked in the urban setting. This area of the brain is active during rumination, which is repetitive thought focused on negative emotions.

120 MINUTES (PER WEEK)

One hundred twenty minutes per week is linked to better overall physical and emotional health. In a 2019 study of 20,000 people, a team led by Mathew White of the European Centre for Environment & Human Health at the University of Exeter found that people who spent two hours a week (either at once or spread out over several visits) in green spaces were substantially more likely to report good health and psychological well-being than those who don't.[58] The effects were robust, cutting across different occupations, ethnic groups, people from rich and poor areas, and people with chronic illnesses and disabilities.

THREE DAYS

From 5- to 120-minute doses, the benefits of time in nature are quite spectacular already. Can you imagine what happens when you spend three full days in nature? In 2012 a group of researchers from the University of Utah and the University of Kansas studied the impact of three days in nature.[59]

The researchers gave tests to 28 backpackers before and after going on their trips. Immediately after a trip, the participants performed 47 percent better in a word-test game that measures creative thinking and insight problem-solving. This improvement and shift in thinking has come to be known as the Three-Day Effect, a term coined by cognitive neuroscientist David Strayer. Strayer hypothesizes that the prefrontal cortex of the backpackers' brains got a much-needed break. Higher-order cognitive functions including selective attention, problem solving, inhibition, and multitasking are all heavily utilized in our modern technology-rich society, and it's hugely beneficial for our brains to get a break every now and again.

Four Steps to Reset Your Relationship with Nature

With the research growing about the benefits of nature and the rise of screen time and the attention economy, we anticipate seeing a lot more nature prescriptions. Of course, one of the best things about a nature prescription is that there are no side effects. It's amazing how much we are willing to put up with when it comes to our more traditional medications for things like anxiety, depression, ADHD, hypertension, and so on.

While it can be helpful and interesting to open ourselves up to the idea that nature is medicine and can be taken in doses, the main takeaway is that *any* amount of nature time is great. Getting a daily dose of nature is one of the most necessary things a person can do to live a healthy, happy, and well-balanced life. For us, this is right up there with eating well, getting quality sleep, exercising, and all the other things we know help us thrive day to day. Here are four steps you can take to start getting your daily, weekly, and monthly doses of nature:

Step 1: Take Nature Breaks (5 minutes)
Step 2: Get your DNA (15 minutes)
Step 3: Go on ENU Adventures (90–120 minutes)
Step 4: Aim for three days every three months (72 hours)

TAKE NATURE BREAKS (5 MINUTES)

Whatever your typical day looks like right now, most of us have the opportunity to take a quick break and to step away and get outside every few hours. And, many of us tend to jump on our phones, computers, or other devices during that time. But the point of a break is to restore, relax, and reenergize. When we go to our devices during that time, we don't give our brains the rest they need! Instead of fitting one more thing in, checking the news, email, or social media feeds, use that time to take a nature break. Remember, just five minutes can boost your mood and positive emotions.

GET YOUR DNA (15 MINUTES)

When we talk about DNA, we're talking about getting our Daily Nature Adventure. By this we mean taking some time—it doesn't have to be long, but we recommend at least fifteen minutes—to experience nature unplugged. Getting your DNA could be as simple as taking a stroll in your local park or green space, doing some urban birding, or going to the beach and putting your feet in the sand and water. The idea here is that this is a relatively simple and accessible way to get our daily dose of nature while mixing in some novelty and adventure. As we learned, spending at least fifteen minutes in nature a day can change our physiology by lowering our cortisol levels (stress), blood pressure, and heart rate.

GO ON ENU ADVENTURES (1½–2 HOURS)

Once a week, find a couple of hours on your calendar to Experience Nature Unplugged (ENU) and go on a mini adventure. These adventures should be just different enough from your daily routine that they create excitement and energy around the experience. They can be relatively short, easy, local, and cheap without skimping on the fun. Adventures can take many forms and be refreshing, rewarding, relaxing, or challenging. Think about a campfire dinner in your backyard, dessert in the park, driving to the mountains or beach to watch a sunset, or finding a new local trail to explore. Find 90–120 minutes on your calendar every week for a mini adventure to reduce depressive symptoms and improve overall physical and psychological health.

AIM FOR THREE DAYS EVERY THREE MONTHS (72 HOURS)

Every three months, try to spend three consecutive days out in nature unplugged. For us, this is typically a weekend camping trip to a relatively local destination (within a couple of hours of where we live). You're certainly welcome to go further or stay longer, but remember that you don't need to go halfway across the globe to do this. The purpose is to bring in the incredible benefits of the Three-Day Effect on a regular basis. We understand that this can be a daunting or challenging task, but the benefits are huge. Whether your limitations are time, money, or access to nature, there are still options to make this a reality. Can't go camping every three months? Consider a nature staycation. Turn off the Wi-Fi, camp in your backyard, and visit a local park or nature space daily. Need to stay connected or on call for work or other responsibilities? Do the best you can to dial up your nature time while managing other obligations. The goal is to get as much nature unplugged time as possible in a three-day period to experience the cognitive benefits of the Three-Day Effect.

More Nature Tips

Nature doses focus on the amount of time spent in nature, which is only part of the equation. How do we actually fit nature time into our day? What will we do when we're outside? What if we don't have easy access to natural or green spaces? These are some of our favorite tips to bring more nature into our lives on a daily basis.

EXPAND YOUR ADVENTURE CIRCLE

Finding a community interested in time in nature is one of the best ways to get outside—and share the work of planning! Find some neighbors who you can share ideas with or partner up with to plan a little excursion.

BRING THE INSIDE OUTSIDE

Are you living most of your life indoors? If so, what activities can be shifted outside (reading, playing games, eating meals)? We tend to get stuck in routines that keep us inside, though many of our daily activities are easy (and sometimes are more fun!) to do outside.

BIRDING

Birding is a great way to connect with nature, and you can do it pretty much anywhere. If you happen to live in the city, urban birding is a great example of how you can get the benefits of nature without going to nature-rich areas or traditional parks. You can open a window or take a walk around the block to experience it.

GET DIRTY

Play in the dirt! It's important to engage our senses when we're out in nature. In fact, it's critical to our tactile and sensory development. Try going barefoot outside, digging in the dirt, climbing trees, or jumping in puddles. This is a great opportunity to channel our distant ancestors, who spent much of their time doing things like digging, climbing, and hunting.

BRINGING THE OUTSIDE INSIDE

Nature can be experienced indoors, too. In addition to getting outside more, there are natural elements you can incorporate in your home to bring nature to you. Consider getting more houseplants for your space. Perhaps start an herb garden in your kitchen or living room window. Maybe even get an oil diffuser and use scents like evergreen or pine to create a calming effect. Air plants are also low maintenance and fun decor. Even things like wood furniture and nature art can change the feel of your space and inspire more time outdoors.

Activity: Four Steps to Reset (in Action)

TAKE NATURE BREAKS (5 MINUTES)

I will fit 5-minute nature breaks into my/our schedules as much as possible:

☐ Before work/school

☐ During lunch
☐ After dinner
☐ In between classes or meetings
☐ When I get home from work/school
☐ _____
☐ _____
☐ _____

To help me achieve this, I will:
    ☐ Put nature breaks on my calendar
    ☐ Find a partner to hold me accountable
    ☐ _____
    ☐ _____
    ☐ _____

GET YOUR DNA (15 MINUTES)
I will find 15 minutes every day for my Daily Nature Adventure.

The best times for my DNA are:
    ☐ Right when I wake up
    ☐ Just before breakfast
    ☐ During lunch
    ☐ After dinner
    ☐ In between classes or meetings
    ☐ Right after work/school
    ☐ Just before bed
    ☐ On the weekends
    ☐ _____
    ☐ _____
    ☐ _____

Activities in support of DNA:
    ☐ Taking a stroll in a local park or nature space
    ☐ Urban birding
    ☐ Dipping my toes in the ocean, lake, river, or creek.
    ☐ Walking barefoot outside
    ☐ Jumping in puddles or climbing trees

☐ Working out outdoors (nature gyms)
☐ _____
☐ _____
☐ _____

To help me achieve this, I will:
☐ Put DNA on my calendar
☐ Find a partner to hold me accountable
   (*Name/s:* _____)
☐ Expand my adventure circle to include
   (*Name/s:* _____)
☐ _____
☐ _____
☐ _____

GO ON ENU ADVENTURES (WEEKLY)

I will go on weekly ENU Adventures that include:
☐ Picnics in the park
☐ Watching the sunset from a new viewpoint
☐ Backyard camping
☐ Sunrise hikes
☐ Neighborhood birding adventures
☐ Ocean dips
☐ Visiting new parks, reserves, or trails
☐ _____
☐ _____
☐ _____

Nature places I have access to and will explore are:
☐ Local parks (*like:* _____)
☐ My backyard and front yard
☐ Nearby nature spaces (*like:* _____)
☐ Beaches (*like:* _____)
☐ _____
☐ _____
☐ _____
☐ _____

To help me achieve this, I will:

- ☐ Put ENU Adventures on my calendar
- ☐ Find a partner to hold me accountable
  (*Name/s:* _____)
- ☐ Expand my adventure circle to include
  (*Name/s:* _____)
- ☐ Embrace the weather and go outside in the rain, wind, cold, heat, or snow
- ☐ _____
- ☐ _____

AIM FOR THREE DAYS EVERY THREE MONTHS

Every three months, I/we will find three days to unplug and immerse in nature by:

- ☐ Taking local camping trips
- ☐ Planning nature-based vacations
- ☐ Turning off Wi-Fi and camping in the backyard
- ☐ Visiting local parks or nature spaces three days in a row
- ☐ _____
- ☐ _____
- ☐ _____

PAUSE AND REFLECT

- *Where in nature did you play as a kid? How did that affect or inspire you?*
- *Connecting with nature is central to our well-being. How do you connect with nature?*

PART THREE

RECONNECT

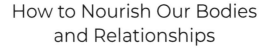

How to Nourish Our Bodies and Relationships

This part of the journey addresses two of the biggest challenges of technology overuse: an increasingly sedentary lifestyle and isolation. Modern technology offers comfort, convenience, and the ability to be connected 24/7. Yet as a society we're sitting more, moving less, and are more isolated and alone than any other time in our history. As a result, we're suffering physically and mentally. To address this, we'll focus on the importance of movement and how to bring more community and connection into our lives. By the end of Part III, we'll have reconnected to our bodies and each other.

CHAPTER 5

Movement

ᘉ

Sitting is the new smoking.
—Dr. James Levine

We're living in an incredible age, with access to technology that makes our lives more convenient and comfortable. However, the countless benefits come with a cost, one of the biggest being our increasingly sedentary lifestyle. With each generation, we are moving less and less. Our parents' generation moved more than ours did, and their parents' generation moved more than they did. Not because we're getting lazier, but because our parents and grandparents had to move out of necessity. Their jobs were often in labor or trade industries and physically intensive. Maintaining the household and associated chores was a full-time job and required significant and continuous movement—and while that still rings true today, many tasks can be done more efficiently with advanced technology. If we go back a few more generations, nearly everyone had a physical role in getting food to the table, whether that was through farming, raising livestock, hunting, or foraging.

Of course, this is not the case anymore. Generally speaking, there is very little that we (in the developed world, particularly in urban settings) have to do in terms of movement. Our household chores are easier, with Roombas (robot vacuums), washing machines, and dishwashers. Few of us farm our own food; in fact, we don't even have to go to the grocery store anymore with apps like DoorDash and Uber Eats. With the click of a button, we can have our favorite meals delivered hot and ready to eat. Online shopping is booming, and we can buy basic necessities, furniture, art and decor, and clothes without leaving the house (or the couch). Much of the workforce has also moved to knowledge-based jobs from labor-intensive or trade-skill work. Movement is minimally required for our day-to-day living and for many has become a leisure activity or a luxury. The World Health Organization (WHO) states that worldwide obesity has nearly tripled since 1975, with a leading cause as "an increase in physical inactivity due to the increasingly sedentary nature of many forms of work, changing modes of transportation, and increasing urbanization."[60]

Earlier we talked about the movie *Wall-E*, where future humans have used up Earth's resources and are living aboard a giant spaceship. Their existence has been taken over by devices and technology. There are so many conveniences built into their lives, like their personal hovercraft vehicles, that they literally have no need to move. As a result, they are soft and round and live most of their lives zooming around in their futuristic little vehicles. Entertainment is built into the screens in front of them, and with a push of a button they can get any food or drink they want. There is an amazing scene where their spaceship tips and all the humans get knocked out of their vehicles. They have been sitting for so long, with no need to use their muscles, that they have trouble standing and moving on their own. Yes, these future humans are a fantasy, but sadly we seem to be heading in that direction.

From a movement perspective, compare humans today (and the imagined *Wall-E* people of the future) to our hunter-gathering ancestors. Hunter-gatherers *had* to move in order to survive. Movement was an integral part of their lives. Whether through exploring, playing, gathering food, hunting, building shelters, or dancing and creating music, movement was continuous throughout their day. Also, consider the incredible *variety* of movement our ancestors had to do on a regular basis compared to us. They had to walk, run, jump, climb, dig, throw, crawl, squat, twist, push, pull, and swim in order to survive. Think about all the different positions they put their bodies in on a daily basis. Now think about your typical day. Maybe life requires a few different twists or squats, but for most of us, movement is optional and the movement we do get takes place within a very limited range of motion. We spend much of our lives sitting, doing things like working on a computer, watching TV, gaming, driving, eating, and socializing.

Much of Sebastian's professional background has been in health and wellness, with a particular focus on movement. He worked as a personal trainer, yoga instructor, and explored a variety of movement modalities for personal and professional interests. A number of years ago, he worked with a company called the Egoscue Method. Their focus is on posture therapy, and they offer clients personalized sequences of exercises tailored to their realignment needs. Working at Egoscue completely reframed his relationship with movement.

A big focus of Egoscue is to encourage movements that are outside the range of our normal, everyday movements. Founder Pete Egoscue describes our lack of movement using an imaginary 2 × 3 foot rectangle that extends from your head to midtorso. Most of our daily movements take place within that box. Activities that make up much of our day, like working at a desk, driving a car, watching TV, cooking a meal, and brushing teeth all happen within a very specific range of motion. We're either sitting and moving in that box or standing and moving in that box. Again, we're typically not doing a lot of twisting, reaching up high, or getting down low or on the ground like our hunter-gatherer ancestors did.

The decrease in the variety of movement and the amount of time we spend moving is staggering. No, we're not advocating a return to a hunter-gatherer lifestyle. The point is to emphasize that we, as humans, need movement to maintain our general well-being, health, and happiness. Since it's hardly required of us these days, we have to be much more intentional about incorporating movement into our lives.

Impact of a Sedentary Lifestyle

As sedentary lifestyles become more common, their impact sometimes becomes less obvious. Statistics can offer powerful and succinct insights. When we look at the stats and the trends—the changes in movement and physical well-being over time—this issue suddenly feels urgent and in need of our immediate attention. Let's take a look.

- Children now spend more than seven and a half hours a day in front of a screen (e.g., TV, video games, computer).[61]
- Nearly one-third of high school students play video or computer games for three or more hours on an average school day.[62]
- More than 80% of adults do not meet the guidelines for both aerobic and muscle-strengthening activities, and more than 80% of adolescents do not do enough aerobic physical activity

to meet the guidelines for youth.[63]

- Recent reports project that by 2030, half of all adults (115 million adults) in the United States will be obese.[64]
- The prevalence of obesity in all age groups, including children, adolescents, and adults, has doubled and in some cases tripled between the 1970s and 2008.[65]
- Between 1998 and 2008 there was a 20% decrease in muscle strength and a 30% decrease in muscle endurance in 10-year-olds.[66]
  - The number of sit-ups 10-year-olds could do declined by 27.1 percent.
  - Arm strength fell by 26 percent and grip strength by 7 percent.
  - While one in 20 children in 1998 could not hold their own weight when hanging from wall bars, one in 10 could not do so in 2008.

Understanding the problem is often helpful and necessary before diving into solutions. Though when we only look at the problem, we're not seeing the entire picture. The problem is what happens when we don't have enough movement in our lives. That's just one side of the coin. The flip side is what happens when we reinsert movement into our lives. Movement elevates mental performance and heightens levels of attention, creativity, focus, and memory. It improves heart and lung function, lowers instances of type 2 diabetes, asthma, high blood pressure, and sleep apnea. Movement also helps build stronger muscles and bones, improves balance, coordination, flexibility, dexterity, and agility.

Benefits of Movement
- Regular exercise improves cardiovascular fitness[67], and reduces blood pressure[68] and blood fat levels.[69]
- Regular aerobic exercise can decrease anxiety[70] and depressive symptoms.[71]
- Exercise can be as effective as medication and psychotherapies for mental health.[72]
- For people with ADHD, a study showed that a single 20-minute

aerobic exercise session improved their symptoms.[73]

- Meditative movement (such as yoga, qigong, tai chi, etc.) has been shown to improve posture, reduce stress, and decrease depressive symptoms and anxiety, leading to a feeling of well-being.[74]
- Synchronized movement (when you move with a group or partner) has been shown to improve self-esteem.[75]
- Walking for 2.5 hours per week (21 minutes per day) can cut your risk of heart disease by 30%.[76]
- Exercise helps build and preserve bone mass.[77]
- Kids with higher levels of fitness score better on standardized tests, especially in math and reading.[78]

Nature Unplugged Movement

Our belief is that any movement is better than no movement, especially in today's digital age. With that said, we want to be very specific here that we're talking about and emphasizing unplugged, outdoor movement similar to that of our hunter-gatherer ancestors. Whether it be a stroll through the park, climbing a tree, or taking a swim in the ocean, getting off our devices and moving in nature is an essential part of overall health and well-being.

When working with our clients, our aim is to help them to incorporate more unplugged outdoor movement into their lives. We're not in the business of prescribing what type of movement people should do. Instead, we work on helping people get in touch with the type of unplugged outdoor movement that works best for them, that they are passionate about and enjoy. Again, any movement is better than no movement. If the only option you have is to jump on a treadmill or stationary bike, it's great to get that movement in. But if there's an opportunity to unplug, incorporate play, and be outside, that's a triple win, and our bodies and minds will thank us for it. Unplugged play can be such a wonderful way to get movement, and there are myriad benefits to doing so. While we will touch on the importance of play briefly in this chapter, we will explore it much further in Chapter 10.

Benefits of Movement in Nature

While we know that movement is wonderful for our minds and

bodies, it's even better when we can get outside and move. In this section we will dive deeper into how awesome it is to exercise in nature. Before we jump into some of the research, think back to our hunter-gatherer ancestors and evolution as a species. We were designed to live, move, and play in connection with the natural world and have spent the vast majority of our time on earth doing just that. It's only been in the very recent past (from an evolutionary perspective) that we have begun spending most of our time indoors, staring at screens.

Even without the research, you've probably had experiences moving in nature that highlighted some of these benefits. Think about your favorite physical activity in nature, whether that's hiking through the woods, swimming in a lake, surfing, skiing, snowboarding, and so on. How do you typically feel beforehand, and then afterward? The fact that moving around outside is good for us isn't new and probably isn't mind-blowing, but it is a helpful reminder. It can be so easy to get sucked into the attention economy (and stuck on the couch) that we have to be more intentional about getting outside and moving.

- Outdoor exercise has been shown to improve mood and reduce depression, beyond that of indoor exercise.[79]
- Walking in nature reduces cortisol, the stress hormone, and increases positive emotions as well as the ability to interact with people positively.[80]
- Exercising in natural, green environments creates greater improvements in adults' self-esteem than exercise in urban or indoor settings.[81]
- Habitual walking in forest environments, but not urban environments, significantly lowered systolic and diastolic blood pressure.[82]
- Exercising outdoors is more psychologically restorative and encourages exercise frequency and consistency.[83]

A 2010 study in the *Journal of Environmental Science and Technology* showed that just five minutes of exercise in a green nature setting can boost mood and self-esteem.[84] Jules Pretty and Jo Barton explain in the study that green exercise is physical activity in the presence of nature. Abundant scientific evidence shows that activity in natural areas decreases the risk of mental illness and improves our sense of well-being. Until now, however, nobody knew how much time people had to spend in green spaces to get those and other benefits.

"For the first time in the scientific literature, we have been able to show dose-response relationships for the positive effects of nature on human mental health," Pretty said. From an analysis of 1,252 people (of different ages, genders, and mental health status) drawn from ten existing studies in the United Kingdom, the authors were able to show that activity in the presence of nature led to mental and physical health improvements.

They analyzed activities such as walking, gardening, cycling, fishing, boating, horse-riding, and farming. The greatest health changes occurred in the young and the mentally ill, although people of all ages and social groups benefited. All natural environments were beneficial, including parks in urban settings. Green areas with water added something extra. A blue and green environment seems even better for health, Pretty noted.

The Importance of Unplugged Movement

We now have a better sense of the benefits of movement, particularly movement in nature. Let's have a look at the importance of "unplugged" movement, where we leave our devices behind. Again, if the only option you have is to get movement in front of a screen, that's better than nothing. But if you can step away from screens and devices and get movement outdoors, that's even better.

When we talk about unplugged movement, we mean taking out the earbuds and taking your eyes off the screen and heading outside. Unplugged movement also means ditching wearable tech (at least occasionally). You don't need to do this every time you exercise, but mixing in some completely unplugged movement has major benefits. Before we get to that, let's spend some time talking about wearable technology.

Part of the wonder and excitement of living in this digital age is access to innovative technology focused on health, wellness, and movement. The market is flooded with devices and gadgets designed to help us learn more about our bodies, how much we move, our sleeping patterns, and all sorts of other things. The amount of information we have access to with a smart watch is amazing. When it comes to wearable tech and gathering data about our movement, there's no doubt that there are some wonderful benefits. We totally get how counting steps or heart rate (or whatever you're interested in measuring) can be helpful in terms of goal setting, motivation, and learning more about your physiology.

While gathering all this information can be helpful, there can also be some drawbacks. One of the challenges is that with so much data feedback, it's difficult to discern what's actually helpful. Similar to the attention economy, it's easy to get sucked into the vortex and rely on our devices and data to see if we're doing well or not. And, just like the attention economy with all its noise, that makes it difficult to be intentional about what we are measuring and why.

One new health trend involves sleep tracking and prompts many of us to check our sleep stats first thing in the morning. Was it a good night's sleep or not? How long did you sleep? How much REM time did you get? How many times did you roll or move or get up to use the bathroom? After reviewing the statistics and going through the morning routine, it's time for the morning workout. The wearable tech is in place and ready, and you begin to move. The stats continue to pour in about heart rate, steps, distance, time, and on and on it goes.

The question to ask at the end of the day is, was that data really helpful and meaningful to my life? If so, what specifically was helpful? Was it all helpful or just certain aspects of it? If your educational background and your work is in exercise science, it could be helpful to have all that information. Without the proper context or education, it may not be so helpful or necessary. In Chapter 3 we explored wellness with technology and the importance of being intentional with the tech in our lives and how we use it. It's the same with wearable technology and what we are measuring. Get in touch with what is really important and helpful and let go of the rest.

Another major drawback of wearable technology is that we often become more focused on the data than what we are actually doing and feeling. We become more interested in a little computer than what our body is telling us. For example, let's say you're doing an intense cardio workout and you're closely tracking and watching your data via smart watch. You notice that your heart rate is higher than normal, so you ease up on the workout even though you feel fine. In fact, you feel great and want to push it harder, but you pull back because of the data. Or, you're feeling really gassed and intuitively know your body needs a rest, but the data suggests you can go harder, so you do.

The issue here is that we are ignoring our bodies' innate intelligence and intuition—an intelligence which has been developing and evolving for thousands of years and is far greater than any smart watch could ever be. Over time we become less in touch with our bodies and more reliant on our devices. Our devices are often a hindrance to being present and mindful when we move. Focusing on our wearable tech takes us out of the moment and out of our direct experience. We lose touch with ourselves and our surroundings.

As an antidote to this, it's key to incorporate unplugged movement into our routine. This doesn't have to be every time you exercise. Again, there is a place for data and gathering information. We recommend doing at least one nature unplugged movement session per week. This could be going to the park or beach (or other natural setting) and doing an activity that helps you experience your surroundings and get in touch with how your body feels. When we incorporate this type of movement, we become more kinesthetically intelligent, and we can cultivate our intuition for the type of movement our bodies are looking for. It's then that we begin to take the power back from our devices and what our tiny computers say we should or shouldn't do. Instead, we intuitively know what's best for ourselves when it comes to movement. Also, when we step back from our devices we are more likely to bring a sense of joy, wonder, and playfulness into our movements.

Sebastian's Story: Nature's Gym

When I first got into the field of health and wellness, I was a personal trainer and yoga instructor. For much of my youth, going to the gym was a huge part of my routine. Throughout high school I would often come home from school and go straight to the beach to surf (if there were waves), followed by a late afternoon or evening gym session. I got a lot of great benefits from going to the gym. I learned a ton about strength training and overall fitness. It was also where I was first introduced to yoga. While there were some great benefits to the gym, there was a part of me that felt disconnected and that something was missing.

It wasn't until later when I was working as a personal trainer and yoga instructor that I really got in touch with what was missing. At this point I was spending much of my time inside the gym and inside the yoga studio. While I enjoyed the work and connecting with my clients, after a while I found myself dulled and bored by the gym environment. It was the same old lighting and the same sounds of cardio machines, television screens, and clinks and clanks from the weights. Most people had headphones on and were locked into the screens on their cardio machines or on the televisions on the walls. Fortunately, there was one gym I worked at which was unique in that it had large windows and great views of a nearby green space. I started to find it strange that day in and day out people (including myself) would be hitting the treadmills, stationary bikes, or lifting weights while looking out at the beautiful scenery rather than going outside to get similar movement.

One day I was working with one of my regular clients. We were just getting started, and I had her doing a warm-up on the treadmill. A few minutes into the warm-up, we were talking about how beautiful a day it was outside. I looked out at the vibrant green grass and majestic willows in the distance. "Hey, Janice, why don't we mix things up and do our warm-up outside today?" She was enthusiastic about the idea. We emerged from the gym and were revitalized by the sunshine and fresh air. We hit the green space and did a light jog around the perimeter. We then mixed things up further and utilized some of the benches and stairs for a variety of strengthening exercises. We ended up having a great session that was a hybrid of indoor and outdoor movement.

That was the beginning of the end of gym life for me. As a personal trainer and yoga instructor, I started to bring more of the outdoors and nature into my work. In my personal workouts I did the same. Instead of hitting the gym, I would go to the beach or local parks and improvise using the natural (and man-made) landscape as my gym. At the beach I could jog, sprint, dig, jump, crawl, and swim. I used the deep sand for running with resistance, or I would run in shallow water. I would jump in the water and swim out through the surf, bodysurf back in to the beach, and repeat. I began to make up my own routines and exercises, and the opportunities were endless. It was the same at the parks. I would use hills and trees and park benches the same ways I used machines in the gym. I'd use playgrounds and monkey bars to climb, pull up, and swing on. This was a total game changer for me. It didn't take me long to realize that I could do nearly everything I did at the gym when I was outdoors.

As I started to see the benefits my clients received in going outdoors, I began taking nearly all of my clients outdoors, whether it was for training or yoga. Over time I began to incorporate other types of nature-based activities. I started to take people hiking, surfing, stand-up paddling, or snorkeling while incorporating aspects of yoga and mindfulness along the way. This shift from the gym to the outdoors was in many ways the origins of Nature Unplugged. It was all about doing mindful movement in nature unplugged.

Tips for Getting More Nature Unplugged Movement

The ideal scenario is to get as much nature unplugged movement as possible in your daily life. You can think of it in tiers of good, better, best. The basic call to action here is to get moving every day, any way you can. Movement is good. What's better is when you can get movement outside or unplug from your devices while you're moving. The absolute best thing you can do for yourself is to find ways to move, be outside in nature, and unplug. Here are some ways to try this out.

TAKE A BREAK FROM WEARABLE TECH

As we have learned, gathering data from our movement can be helpful, but it can also be a hindrance. Make it a weekly goal to spend at least one day per week without any wearable tech. This is a great way to mix things up, bring more mindfulness into your day/exercise, and to get in touch with your body's innate intelligence and intuition.

JOIN NATURE'S GYM

Instead of going to the gym and hitting the treadmill, go for a walk or run outside. Get creative with your workouts around the neighborhood and at the park by utilizing nature and natural resources as workout equipment. There are so many wonderful options—you can make use of the trees, rocks, or benches and tables. Also, consider leaving your wearable tech at home every now and then. While counting steps and receiving data feedback can be helpful, it can also take away from the experience. Even if it's not practical or appropriate to cancel your gym membership and go full-on Tarzan, we do highly encourage you to vary your indoor routine by using nature as a gym from time to time.

EMBRACE THE WEATHER

It may seem easiest to enjoy the outdoors when there's sunshine and warmth, but cold, rain, and snow can bring nature to life in a totally new way. They also open the door to a different set of activities. Playing in the rain and jumping in puddles can be delightful at any age. The damp ground brings new bugs and insects out to explore and admire. With snow comes sledding, snow angels, snowmen, and snowball fights. Weather is something to be embraced, not avoided. When the seasons change, or a storm comes through, consider it a call to adventure. For a little cold weather outdoor exercise motivation, check out https://www.wimhofmethod.com.

MOVE WITHOUT YOUR PHONE

For example, many of us bring our phones with us on a walk by habit. But what do you need it for? A typical walk in the neighborhood or local nature space is relatively safe, and unless you're waiting for an important call, it's hard to see why you *need* your phone with you. When you leave your phone at home, you'll be less distracted and more immersed in your movement. You'll start to notice the weather, the bugs and birds, the houses and trees, and the other people who are also out for a walk. As much as possible, get outside and leave your phone at home.

GET OUT OF THE BOX

Most of our movement takes place within an imaginary two-foot-wide by three-foot-high box right in front of us. Remember to get outside the box regularly throughout your day. Stand up and stretch your hands to the sky, get down on the floor and crawl around. There are so many different ways to do this, and the more you can get outside the box, the better.

JOIN A TEAM

Great movement, accountability, and a chance to socialize are a few of the perks of joining a rec league or team. Most areas have a variety of leagues that offer things like kick ball, soccer, tennis, pickleball, flag football, and volleyball. You can create your own team, sign up with a small group, or solo as a free agent.

MOVE HOW YOU WANT

Sometimes it feels like the options and opportunities for movement available to adults are limited and boring. Life's too short to spend time doing things you don't enjoy when there are alternatives available. If you don't like running but enjoy the cardio, try dancing, jumping rope, or hula hooping and see if it hits the spot. The goal is to find a way to move around that works for you, because if you enjoy it, you'll keep doing it.

Activity: Reconnecting to Our Bodies

Remember, any movement is better than no movement. But the absolute best thing we can do to counter the effects of sitting in front of screens all day is to find ways to move our bodies, be outside in nature, and unplug.

I commit to getting _____ minutes/hours of movement every day.

To help me achieve this, I will:
- [ ] Put movement on my calendar
- [ ] Use nature as my gym
- [ ] Go on a walk without my phone
- [ ] Get out of the box with big stretches and crawling
- [ ] Embrace the weather (instead of using it as an excuse)
- [ ] Take breaks from wearable tech
- [ ] _____
- [ ] _____
- [ ] _____

PAUSE AND REFLECT

- *What types of movement do you enjoy most?*
- *What new physical activities have you been wanting to try?*
- *What challenges or competing priorities keep you from getting the amount of movement and physical activity you want?*
- *What small shifts can you make to get closer to your movement goals?*

CHAPTER 6

Community and Connection

The opposite of addiction is not sobriety.
It is human connection.

—Johann Hari

Two of the greatest challenges of living in the digital age are increasingly sedentary lifestyles and isolation. In the last chapter we addressed our sedentary lifestyle and focused on movement and reconnecting to our bodies. Now, let's explore how we can reconnect to each other and our communities in more meaningful ways.

The Case for Connection

In his riveting book *Chasing the Scream*, journalist Johann Hari takes readers on a journey into the origins of the drug war and sheds light on what really causes addiction and what really solves it.[85] The book tells a different story from what many of us are familiar with. Rather than addiction being largely caused by a chemical hook and weak morals, Hari explores how factors like childhood trauma, social isolation, and a lack of engaged living can play a huge role in addiction. He makes a convincing case that the opposite of addiction is human connection.

While this book isn't about drug addiction, some of the same contributing factors are at work in our relationships with technology. Our view is that a big part of the solution is similar to what Hari uncovered in his research. The long-term solution to negative effects from tech overuse are things like connection and engaged living. We're talking about connection to nature, connection to ourselves, and connection to other humans, to our community. Human connection isn't in the category of "nice to have." It's a "must-have," and is essential for us as social creatures.

In *Chasing the Scream*, Hari details how we've been treating drug addicts in the country, and around most of the world, for the past one hundred or so years since the war on drugs began. Addicts have been severely punished; they've been locked up, isolated, humiliated, and in many cases when they do attempt to reengage with society, their records make it very difficult to find meaningful work. It's important to point out that his book isn't condoning drug use or advocating it. Hari's research simply shows that this treatment of addicts and addiction doesn't do much to solve the problem of addiction. In fact, this only perpetuates the issue. People who are isolated and aren't engaged in society are much more likely to go back to using various substances.

It's interesting to note that in our society we are seeing a similar thing happen, for completely different reasons, of course. Instead of being locked away and isolated for illegal drug use, many of us are voluntarily isolating and locking ourselves away out of convenience and comfort, largely as a result of advances in technology. To clarify, it's not so much that we are voluntarily isolating ourselves but that the attention economy is so powerful it's encouraging us to spend more time alone glued to our devices. A thought-provoking comparison from Edward Tufte exemplifies this: "There are only two industries that call their customers 'users': illegal drugs and software."

We've talked about these conveniences throughout this book. We have pretty much everything we need at our fingertips. Our smartphones can provide entertainment, information, education, access to social media, and food-ordering with just a few clicks. It's amazing! And, as we've discussed before, there's a downside. Because there is often no need to leave the comfort and safety of our home, we're spending more and more time in our own little bubbles. One of the side effects of this is that we've become the most sedentary humans in history. More on that in the next chapter.

We're seeing huge trends of voluntary isolation as a society. More people are working from home. More young people come straight home after school and stay home on weekends to play video games, surf the web, watch YouTube, etc. More of our social life and sense of community is moving to virtual spaces (and not just for young people and millennials). The 2020 COVID-19 pandemic only forced this trend further.

Just like in *Chasing the Scream*, the more we become isolated and cut off from our tribes and sense of community, the less healthy we are physically and mentally. This is certainly a contributing factor in the rise of mental health issues in our culture, such as anxiety, depression, and myriad other problems. Many of these issues would be resolved with more of an emphasis on human connection and community.

Talking to Strangers

As a social species, one of the harshest things you can do to humans is put them in total isolation. Solitary confinement in prisons is for the worst offenders. While we know isolation is harmful, an interesting paradox takes place with commuters around the world every day. People are moving from place to place on buses, trains, and subways, sitting inches away from each other, and they often actively ignore each other. Observe the dynamics of pretty much any commuting system in the developed world and you'll see a lot of screens, headphones, and downward stares.

Of course, you could make the case that this dynamic isn't just a result of the digital age and that commuters were doing the same thing prior to the release of the smartphone. Instead of phones, people kept their heads buried in books, magazines, and newspapers. While this is true, it's also very different today because of the attention economy. The analog items had natural pauses, magazines came to an end, and you had to put your book or newspaper away before getting up and exiting the train. Today, social media and news scrolls are never-ending, and many of us continue to read the news, skim our emails, or listen to podcasts while we walk off the train.

To see what the psychological effects were of commuters engaging with others versus keeping to themselves, University of Chicago Business School researchers Nicholas Epley and Juliana Schroeder looked at this paradox of commuting in a 2014 study.[86] The researchers examined commuters on the 'L' trains in Chicago and grouped people in one of three conditions. Group one was put in a connection condition, and they were asked to engage in conversation with other people during their commute. The second group was put in an isolation condition, and people were instructed not to talk to anyone and keep to themselves. The third group was the control group, and they were asked to go about their business as usual, doing what they normally would do during their commute. Each group had their well-being measured at the end of the train ride and end of the day to see what the impact was.

Before the subjects embarked on their commutes, they were asked what they thought would happen and to predict the outcome. As you might have guessed, the group in the solitude condition thought they would enjoy their time alone, and the group in the connection condition thought it would be awkward to connect and talk with strangers, resulting in a lower well-being. What they found was the opposite of their predictions. People in the solitary condition dropped below baseline, and those in the connection condition reported a big boost in positivity.

This study has been replicated across a number of cities and spaces with similar results. What a wonderful reminder to put our devices down and engage with those around us. One of the biggest takeaways is the reminder that what we think is going to be beneficial to us often isn't. This is especially true when it comes to community and connection. It's easy to think we'll feel better in keeping to ourselves, in staying home and avoiding others, when in reality this often makes us feel worse.

Failure to Thrive

One of the biggest factors involved in living well in the digital age is our ability to stay connected physically. The COVID-19 pandemic amplified challenges around connection in that it required physical distance between people and discouraged touch. In the United States and across the world, mental health challenges rose significantly during the pandemic, and it's reasonable to link those increases to lost connection, separation from friends, family, our community, and general isolation.

We can look to a series of studies done in the early part of the twentieth century for more information about the negative effects isolation has on humans. In the early 1900s, the mortality rates of infants placed in orphanages, nurseries, and foundling hospitals were extremely high. In some cases the rate was close to 100%. And, of the babies who didn't die, many of them grew up with all sorts of physical and psychological issues. These babies had all they needed in terms of food and medicine, but they were missing something critical: human touch and human affection. During this time there was much less human connection and physical contact in orphanages and nurseries. Nurses were required to wear face masks and the family was kept separated from newborns to prevent the spread of disease and infection. In the 1940s researchers started to look at this issue. Dr. Henry Bawkin, who was one of the first physicians to research this condition, said, "failure of infants to thrive in institutions is due to emotional deprivation."[87]

Fortunately, this research and new understanding regarding the importance of touch and connection led to big changes in medical protocols that decreased infant mortality rates. There continues to be a great deal of research conducted on the importance of skin-to-skin touch with infants. It's interesting to compare what was happening with infants in the first part of the twentieth century with what's happening now. We are spending less time with each other and more time alone with our devices. The comfort and conveniences technological advances have given us tend to promote virtual connection in virtual spaces. Yet the science shows that the absence of touch, affection, and physical, in-person connection comes at a cost. So, we need to pay extra attention in our high-tech world to finding ways to connect with others.

Cultivating Connection

It's important to understand the impact of being isolated and disconnected from our fellow humans. Knowing its effects gives us a platform as we move to change our reality. It gives us a reason to want something different and seek it. Two of the most meaningful ways to cultivate deeper connections are (1) striving for a higher quality of communication and (2) understanding that feelings follow behaviors.

AIM FOR HIGHER QUALITY OF COMMUNICATION

One of the wonders of the digital age is all the ways we can communicate with each other. There are so many different options, it's incredible. We can "like" something on social media, we can send emojis, we can text, we can talk on the phone, we can do video calls, and we can go old school and talk in person, just to name a few. There are lots of options, but not all of them are created equal. When it comes to building connection and community, some are more effective than others. It can be helpful to think of the quality of communication in terms of the amount of information and data that is available to us. The higher the quality of communication, the more information we can collect; the lower the quality of communication, the less information there is.

Cal Newport, author of *Digital Minimalism*, brought the practice of minimizing digital clutter and distraction mainstream.[88] He spends considerable time in his book discussing the importance of reclaiming real-world, in-person conversation. In fact, Newport has an entire chapter dedicated to this, titled "Don't Click 'Like.'" We agree with that advice and consider social media "likes" to be on the lower end of the communication spectrum. There is not a ton of information we can gather from a like and there is not a ton of actual connection happening. Just above "likes" are things like emojis and memes, then come text messages and emails. A phone call is another step up. With a phone call, you can have a flowing conversation and can pick up on all sorts of information that's not available through written text. You can gather additional information from the tone of someone's voice, their inflections, pauses, and energy level. All of this helps us to feel heard and connect more genuinely to another person. A video call is a big step up from a phone call. Not only is there free-flowing conversation and access to words and tone of voice, but we can also visually pick up on facial expressions and body language.

Often cited in communication research is the psychologist Albert Mehrabian. He is most well known for his work on effective communication and the use of nonverbal and paraverbal messages. According to Mehrabian, verbal messages—the words we say—account for only 7% of the information shared and received. Our tone, pitch, and the pace of our voice—paraverbal messages—account for 38% of our communication, and the final 55% is made up of our nonverbal messages—eye contact, facial expressions, body language. If we think of communicating with each other as message senders and receivers, more information (verbal + nonverbal + paraverbal) translates to a more complete message. That means the highest quality of communication you can get is an undistracted, in-person, face-to-face, old-fashioned conversation.

In-person communication also allows for immediate feedback. We hear words spoken out loud with tone and inflection—we can see the person's face, his or her posture and overall body language; we have access to other sensory information, like smell and touch—and we can adjust our message in real time based on the other person's nonverbal and paraverbal feedback. It has the highest potential for a quality connection because it yields the most information and is dynamic. Face-to-face interactions are shown to produce higher levels of satisfaction with the social experience, a higher degree of closeness to one another, and a deeper level of self-disclosure.[89]

However, having an in-person, face-to-face, undistracted conversation is not always possible, especially in this day and age. The key is to aim for the highest form of communication that you can, given your resources and circumstances. There is a time and place for likes, emojis, memes, and texts. The important thing to recognize is that likes and emojis don't create or allow for the type of connection that we need as human beings. In other words, "liking" 100 of your friend's posts on social media still falls significantly short of a quick phone call or coffee date, both in terms of the quality of communication and connection. In fact, researchers and psychologists like Sherry Turkle (2015) argue that our increasing shift to digital communication over face-to-face conversation isn't just a less rich form of communication; it's splitting our attention and diminishing our overall capacity for empathy.[90]

SONYA AND SEBASTIAN'S STORY: LONG-DISTANCE CONNECTION

Sonya and I first met in Barcelona, Spain. Sonya happened to be my sister's housemate. They were enrolled in the same work and study program in Spain to teach English as a foreign language. My sister had been living in Barcelona for about six months, and I had made plans to visit her for the winter holidays. My family visit ended up getting a little sidetracked after meeting Sonya. To make a long story short, we ended up hitting it off, and out of nowhere started a long-distance relationship. Neither of us intended to get into a distance relationship, but crazy things can happen when love gets into the mix.

At the time, I was traveling extensively, leading surfing and yoga retreats abroad. So, although San Diego was my home base, any relationship would have had a bit of distance with the amount of traveling I was doing. Sonya had just finished graduate school and had set off to Spain to mix things up before her plan of returning to the U.S. to work in higher education. I don't think she was planning on meeting an American while she was in Spain, but perhaps it was part of her plan all along.

Not long after we first met in Barcelona, we set up our second rendezvous in Morocco, where I would be for a surf retreat. After having an amazing time in Marrakech, we were able to work it out so that we saw each other in person every few months. While this wasn't too hard initially, as time went on, those spaces in between in-person meetings became more and more difficult. Fortunately, with the amazing advances in digital communication, we were able to stay in touch via text and phone conversations. But what really was a game changer (and in my opinion, a relationship saver) was the ability to video chat. We had weekly "dates" via video chat, and it was amazing how connected we were able to stay through that medium. Being able to not only hear her words and tone but see her facial expressions and body language was incredible. Not only were we able to sustain our relationship, but we were also able to build on it during that time.

Of course, video chat paled in comparison to our in-person, face-to-face time together, but I don't know that we'd be where we are today without it. Thankfully, after a little over a year of distance and mostly digital communication, we were able to find a way to be together in person in San Diego. While I'm happy those days of the distance relationship are behind us, I do look back on those times fondly and am deeply grateful for the technology that helped us stay connected when we were physically so far apart.

FEELINGS FOLLOW BEHAVIORS

Think back to the study about talking to strangers on a train. Remember how the participants predicted that they'd be less happy interacting with other people than if they were to sit quietly by themselves? It's such an interesting paradox and something we've all probably experienced. Even with the intellectual understanding that social interactions are good for us, it can be challenging to put ourselves out there and initiate conversations and connection, especially with strangers. One concept that can be helpful to explore is that feelings follow behaviors.

This means that we often need to step into the behavior (action) first, and then the feelings and emotions follow. A great example of this is exercise. Many of us wait until we feel ready and excited to work out before we actually go work out. In this case, we are expecting and waiting for the feelings to come before the behavior. We often don't feel quite up to it, finding excuses like "It's been a long day" or "I didn't sleep that well last night," and we don't end up exercising. Sound familiar? On the flip side, when we understand that the feeling will follow the behavior, we know the good feelings and motivation come after we get moving. With a little push, we can move ourselves into action, and then everything changes.

The same thing happens when it comes to human connection. If we wait until we're really feeling perky and social in order to reach out to our fellow humans, whether they are friends or strangers, it probably isn't going to happen. The couch and Netflix, social media, our emails and work, or the news begin to pull us in. But, if we can recognize and remind ourselves that feelings follow behavior, we can reach out first, knowing that the good feelings—positive emotions and a sense of connection—will follow.

Community and Connection Tips

Similar to other concepts and ideas, when it comes to building community and connection, an intellectual understanding of these principles only goes so far. These concepts are only helpful if we can put them into action. The following tips are some of our favorite ways to step into connection.

REDEFINE QUALITY TIME

Couples, friends, and families can get into ruts where it feels like we're all just going through the motions. Work to set the scene for your time together to prime it for a high quality of connection. Ditch your devices and plan an evening without digital distractions. Do something novel and new. Get a set of table topic cards to guide your conversation into new terrain. Cook a new meal together. Hike a new trail. Stargaze. Maybe even break out a few of your favorite board games.

FIND A MEETUP GROUP

Finding a group of people who share your interests is a great way to bring a sense of community into your life. Meetup groups take many forms and cover a wide range of activities, like sports, religion, food, wine, and books. If you're new to an area, or your current friends don't share a specific interest of yours, go find folks who do! And, if it doesn't already exist, create a new group yourself.

VOLUNTEER

Helping others, especially those in our community, is often incredibly rewarding. This can take many forms, like beach, park or road cleanups, serving at soup kitchens, repairing run-down spaces, fences or buildings, delivering groceries, or helping fundraisers. Volunteering engages us more deeply with others in our community whom we are otherwise less likely to interact with on a daily basis.

TALK TO STRANGERS

Challenge yourself to talk to at least one stranger every day. Whether you're at a Starbucks, on the bus, out for a walk, in the elevator, or waiting in a checkout line, push yourself to say hello and ask an open-ended question.

SKIP THE SELF-CHECKOUT LINES

Even if you've only got two things in your basket, check out in a line with the cashier. Sure, it's nice to fly through the self-checkout line at times, but it's a missed opportunity for human contact and connection. Over the course of a day, these missed opportunities can add up, especially as more services become automated. Strike up a conversation with the cashier—ask about weekend plans or his or her opinion about a product you're buying.

TOUCH AND AFFECTION: HUMANS AND PETS

OK, let's be clear that we're talking about consensual and appropriate touch and affection. Hug your friends and family, cuddle, or hold hands. Touch is critical to our well-being, so make the most of what's available to you. If you live alone and aren't able to see friends or family often, consider getting a pet. We can create meaningful relationships, connection, and even a sense of community with our pets.

Activity: Connection Over Comfort and Convenience

RECONNECTING TO OTHERS

I will prioritize social connection over comfort and convenience by:

- ☐ Joining a Meetup group
- ☐ Signing up for a rec league
- ☐ Starting or joining a book club
- ☐ Talking to a stranger every day
- ☐ Skipping the self-checkout line
- ☐ Hugging friends and family
- ☐ Cuddling with my partner
- ☐ Getting a pet
- ☐ _____
- ☐ _____
- ☐ _____

AIM FOR A HIGHER QUALITY OF COMMUNICATION

Whenever possible, I will prioritize the quality of my communication over comfort and convenience by:

- ☐ Putting my phone away when I'm with friends or family
- ☐ Calling instead of texting when I have the time
- ☐ Sharing important news in person
- ☐ Reaching out directly instead of checking a social media page for updates
- ☐ _____
- ☐ _____
- ☐ _____

PAUSE AND REFLECT

- *What's the single biggest change you could make in your relationships—the way you connect and engage with others and your community?*
- *What are you going to change? How? When? Make a quick plan to put it into action.*

PART FOUR

REWIRE

How to Strengthen Our Awareness, Build Resilience, and Live in Alignment with Our Values

It may be helpful to think of the earlier parts of this book as the tangible fixes that set us on the right path and get us out of our own way. We call them technical solutions. If "Reset" and "Reconnect" are the tip of the iceberg, then "Rewire" is about diving beneath the surface and doing the deeper and more adaptive work. This part is all about building and strengthening your inner force field against the attention economy. Doing this inner work opens us up to new possibilities and will help ensure that we don't get pulled back into old patterns. By the end of Part IV, we will have rewired how we think, approach challenges, deal with disappointment, celebrate successes, and cultivate curiosity.

CHAPTER 7

Mindfulness

∿

Breathe.
You are alive!
—Thich Nhat Hanh

Now that we understand the challenges of living in the digital age, have our tech boundaries in place, and are bringing more nature, movement, and connection into our lives, it's time to dive deeper. To begin, we will look at the practice of mindfulness as a way to be more intentional every day.

What does mindfulness mean to you? What words, concepts, or practices come to mind? You may think of things like walking in the woods on a beautiful morning listening to birds chirping all around you. You may think of practices like yoga and tai chi. You may connect mindfulness with religion or spirituality. You may have a positive relationship with it or you may be averse to it. You may think of mindfulness as a fad or as something you should do but don't want to or don't have the time to. People often equate mindfulness with other words and concepts, like attention, presence, awareness, alertness, being, and consciousness. If, for whatever reason, the word "mindfulness" doesn't resonate with you, we encourage you to replace it with a word that works better for you.

Whether you're familiar with mindfulness or new to it, our aim for this chapter is to (1) help make mindfulness useful and relevant in day-to-day life, (2) explore why it plays such a vital role in creating healthy relationships with technology and nature, and (3) show how you can enjoy the benefits of formal and informal mindfulness practices regardless of religious or spiritual beliefs.

What is Mindfulness?

If you search for a definition of mindfulness, you'll find many different options. There are so many that it can quickly become confusing. In order for us to all be on the same page, we're going to go with the definition by scientist and mindfulness researcher Jon Kabat-Zinn. Kabat-Zinn defines mindfulness as "paying attention in a particular way: on purpose, in the present moment, and nonjudgmentally."

We're using this definition because it's clear, succinct, and simply put. Mindfulness is the practice of intentionally bringing our attention (focus) to the present moment in a nonjudgmental way. Mindfulness, in its essence, is a recognition that the only moment we ever actually experience is right now, this present moment. And, that we are often pulled out of the present moment by thoughts of the future or thoughts of the past. Thoughts about the future are fantasies and thoughts about the past are memories.

The concept of mindfulness is simple in theory, but is often quite challenging to put into practice. Understanding the concept, however, isn't very helpful *unless* it's put into practice. We want to emphasize the word "practice" here. It's important to make the transition from mindfulness being a concept that we intellectually understand to a practice and a way of being in the world, from moment to moment.

Mindfulness ... So Hot Right Now

Published Mindfulness Articles (goAMRA.org)

Mindfulness is now hip and in the mainstream. At the time of writing this, if you google mindfulness, you'll get 250 million results. With mindfulness hashtags and yoga pictures, mindfulness seems to be everywhere—a quick search or scroll on social media will show you just how popular it is. Stories on mindfulness are constantly in the news and in magazines. In 1996, three articles written about mindfulness appeared in scientific journals. By 2007, three became 69, and by 2016, there were 667 articles published. As we like to say, mindfulness ... it's so hot right now.

While the concept of mindfulness has gone viral, it's important to note that the practice of mindfulness is not new. In fact, it's ancient, though tracing its roots is difficult. Some historians point to the ancient practice of yoga as the origin of a formal mindfulness practice, which can be traced back more than 5,000 years. Some researchers even think that yoga may be up to 10,000 years old. Many connect the practice of mindfulness to Buddhism, which began more than 2,500 years ago. While the roots of mindfulness are often traced back to ancient India, mindfulness is not specific to any culture, religion, race, or civilization.

So, how did mindfulness become so popular in the West? Jon Kabat-Zinn, whose definition we used, played a big role in bringing the practice of mindfulness to the Western world. Kabat-Zinn, a researcher and longtime practitioner of mindfulness and meditation, was interested in finding a way to study the impact of mindfulness practice. In the 1970s he created a program called Mindfulness-Based Stress Reduction (MBSR) to do just that. The purpose of this eight-week program was to give participants a foundational understanding of mindfulness in theory and (more importantly) practice. The program also stripped away many of the religious and spiritual aspects of the practice, allowing scientists to study the impact of mindfulness through research.

The program was a success and opened the door for mindfulness to take hold in the West. The research that came out of the MBSR programs showed that mindfulness did have measurable positive effects on participants. Suddenly mindfulness moved from a nice-sounding concept to a practice with tangible benefits. Since the 1970s there has been extensive research on the benefits of practicing mindfulness, and more is piling up.

A Force Field from the Attention Economy

There are countless measurable benefits to mindfulness. A number of studies out of Harvard show that mindfulness prevents an array of physical and mental conditions, including irritable bowel syndrome, fibromyalgia, psoriasis, anxiety, depression, and post-traumatic stress disorder.[91] It's an evidence-based practice for reducing stress and anxiety. Additionally, research has found that the practice has been shown to lower blood pressure and even create changes in our genes.[92]

At Nature Unplugged, we view the practice of mindfulness as foundational to developing healthy relationships with technology and nature. Mindfulness is also our best defense against the attention economy. We've been teaching mindfulness practices to our clients in our coaching, workshops, and retreats over the years because we know it works. At its core, it is about building our capacity to pay attention and move through our day with intention. As we have learned (thanks to the attention economy), there are a lot of companies whose sole aim is to capture our attention and keep it for as long as possible. Without a practice of mindfulness, without intentionality, we are at the whim of the attention economy and the tech in our lives. Without mindfulness, we are like a ship without an anchor, floating about at the mercy of the wind and ocean currents.

Just like going to the gym and lifting weights helps build our muscles and strength, practicing mindfulness helps build our "muscles" of attention. Once we've built our muscles of attention, we will be more intentional and aware of how and when we are using technology. We will be less prone to distraction and being pulled into the tech vortex. (That's when you pull out your phone for a second to check the weather, but also end up looking at emails, texts, and social media feeds; then, 30 minutes later, you come to your senses and wonder what happened.) With mindfulness, that happens less and less frequently, and eventually we can avoid the tech vortex altogether.

Similarly, mindfulness is key to developing our relationship with nature. Paying attention to our thoughts, feelings, and to the physical sensations of our body can be key to understanding when we need to take a break from our screens and devices and go outside. It is typically when we are not mindful that we go for extended periods of time without experiencing nature unplugged.

Let's say you have a fifteen-minute break at work. It's easy to jump on your phone to check the news or social media without giving it much thought. With mindfulness, we have the option of doing something different. We have the ability to more clearly get in touch with what we want. If we want to spend our break checking the news and our social media feed, that's one thing. The problem is when this behavior (pulling out our phones to check the news or social media) becomes automatic and unintentional. With mindfulness, we can check in with ourselves and consider if we want to check our phone or perhaps go for a walk around the building or sit near some trees. With mindfulness, we have options and are much more likely to opt to choose nature.

The wonderful thing about mindfulness is that it's not only good for your mental and physical well-being, it's hugely beneficial in being more intentional with technology and nature, and it can also be used as a way to boost performance. It's being practiced in a wide variety of areas, including athletics and business. Many top professional athletes and teams incorporate mindfulness into their routine and philosophy. Legendary basketball coach Phil Jackson used yoga and meditation to improve his team's performance.[93] In the NFL, Seattle Seahawks coach Pete Carroll and sports psychologist Michael Gervais incorporate a wide variety of mindfulness practices into their training and game preparation.[94] There are also a number of top executives (especially in the tech world) who practice mindfulness as a way to increase performance and mental clarity in their very demanding positions.

Mindfulness in Nature

While there are many different options for practicing mindfulness, our very favorite way is to unplug and get outside. As we explored in the last chapter, nature has an amazing way of engaging our senses and grabbing our attention. We look at unplugged time in nature as a mindfulness practice. Whether you're feeling the bumps and ridges of the earth beneath your feet on a mountain trail, listening to the birds chirping in the trees high above, or smelling the fragrance of the pines, it's all mindfulness. And when you practice mindfulness in nature, it's a win-win. Not only do you get all the benefits of being out in nature (as we discussed in the last chapter), but you get all the benefits of mindfulness as well. How awesome is that? In the following story, Sebastian shares how spending time in nature (and listening to bird calls in particular) can be a great way to bring more mindfulness into your life.

Sebastian's Story: Can You Hear the Hummingbirds?

If I were to claim to have a superpower, it would be this: I can hear hummingbirds nearly all the time ... at least when I'm outside, when it's daytime, and when I'm in San Diego or some other happening hummingbird spot. They seem to follow me around, and it's awesome!

I think about hummingbirds often, and the little buzzing beings have been a major source of inspiration over the years. Hummingbird encounters at my favorite local park are what inspired me to write *The Adventures of Enu*.[95] I look at hummingbirds as little reminders to be present. There have been countless times I've been out mindlessly walking, and then out of nowhere comes the peculiar call of the hummingbird to wake me up again.

A few years ago, when I was just getting into leading surf and yoga retreats internationally, I found myself overwhelmed by all the things I had to do to get ready for an upcoming trip. At the time I was working with a great friend, professional surfer John Maher. We were gearing up to take a group of people down to Nicaragua for a ten-day trip. Doing this type of work had always been my dream, though I suppose I never realized how much goes into facilitating a retreat. I had so many things on my mind: finding accommodation, working out all the finances, arranging flights from different cities, getting all the surf gear ready, checking the weather and surf forecasts, arranging transportation and meals. The list went on and on.

I found myself overwhelmed and desperately needing a break from all the tasks at hand. So, I headed over to my favorite park for a quick stroll. As I drove to the park, I was lost in thought. Have you ever driven somewhere and then upon arrival wondered how you got there because you had almost no recollection of the drive? Well, that was my experience on this particular day. I got out of my car and set out on an afternoon stroll around the beautiful park.

I went past the duck pond and on to the hiking trail. I meandered through the coastal sage scrub and oak trees as I normally do. I had been walking for probably twenty minutes before it hit me. I hadn't heard a single hummingbird, or bird for that matter, since entering the park! This particular park happens to be a total hummingbird mecca (my opinion), and I typically hear one within the first couple of minutes. *What was going on? What happened to the hummingbirds?* I wondered. At the moment I began to question what was going on, I realized I had been so consumed with thoughts and worries, to-do lists, and arrangements regarding the Nicaragua trip that I had completely missed out on my walk. I was so focused on the upcoming trip and my internal dialogue was so "noisy" that I was hardly aware of anything else.

With that realization, my internal chatter began to quiet as if someone had turned down a dimmer switch. As my mind quieted down, the sounds of the birds chirping and cheeping began to flow in. A moment later, I heard the high-pitched call of the mighty hummingbird. I smiled as I watched the tiny bird dart overhead. I then looked around at my surroundings. The colors of the trees and flowers were suddenly vibrant with life. Of course, the beauty and the birds had been there the whole time, but I hadn't been there for them. I was too busy thinking about where I was going to be.

That day stands out to me as a reminder to ask myself, *Can I hear the hummingbirds?* This reminder has really helped improve my skills at locating hummingbirds. More importantly, however, it's helped me bring more attention to life as it unfolds moment by moment. It's helped me bring that quality of awareness to listening to myself, other people, and to the world around me. Regardless of my surroundings or what I'm doing, I've made it a habit to ask myself, Can I hear the hummingbirds? When I ask this simple question, it changes the quality of my communication, my relationships, and my life.

Types of Mindfulness Practices

Now that we have a sense of what mindfulness is, where it comes from, and why it's important, let's look at some different types of practices. The great news is that there are lots of different ways to practice mindfulness and incorporate it into your life. Like many things, there is no one-size-fits-all. The key is finding the practice that works best for you and approaching it with the beginner's mind.

The beginner's mind is essentially just what it sounds like: engaging in a practice or a task from the perspective of a beginner. When you approach something from the mindset of a beginner, you are open and receptive to all the possibilities, things are new and exciting, and there's a spirit of play in what you do. The opposite would be to approach something from the perspective of the expert. From the expert's point of view, there is nothing left to learn and the possibilities are few. Of course, you can be very experienced—or expert—at something and still approach it with a beginner's mind. Think about professional athletes like Argentine footballer (soccer player) Lionel Messi. He's clearly an expert at his craft, yet he brings a spirit of playfulness and creativity to the game that is novel and fresh. So, whether you're new to mindfulness or have been practicing it for years, it's a helpful reminder to approach this with a beginner's mind.

Mindfulness is often divided into two types of practices: formal and informal. Formal practices are when we engage in an intentional, structured mindfulness activity for a set amount of time. For example, a 30-minute yoga practice every morning. There are many different types of formal practices: breathing meditation, body scan, eating meditation, walking meditation, yoga, tai chi, and so on. Informal practices, on the other hand, are everything outside of one's formal practice. Practicing mindfulness informally is how you bring present-moment awareness into your day-to-day activities, such as washing dishes, driving a car, talking with friends, working, and so on.

The formal and informal practices build off of each other. To use a sports metaphor, think of the formal practice of mindfulness like practicing the fundamentals of soccer. It's key to practice and develop skills like ball control, dribbling, passing, and shooting. When you have practiced the fundamentals, they are much easier to apply during game time, which of course will not only make you a better player but will also make the game more enjoyable. Eventually, you don't even have to think about the fundamentals during game time because you know them so well (and because you continue to practice). It's the same thing with mindfulness; when you practice the fundamentals (formal practice), it's much easier to use those skills in day-to-day life (the game), especially when things get challenging.

Developing a formal practice of mindfulness is one of the key ways to cultivate wellness in the digital age. In the appendix we have provided brief descriptions and instructions for four formal mindfulness practices to explore: a breathing meditation, a body scan, an eating meditation, and a walking meditation. This is by no means an exhaustive list of options. The idea is to give you a feel for some of the different practices as a foundation to build on. While it's important to incorporate the formal practices on a regular basis, it's more important to be able to bring the practice of mindfulness into everyday activities.

Activity: Mindfulness in Nature

Increase your presence outdoors by engaging your senses with this four-part challenge. Pick a day this week to spend some time outside in a nature setting. This could be a park, the beach, or just outside your front or back door. Whatever you have access to will work great. Remember, the benefits of nature can be felt in just a few minutes!

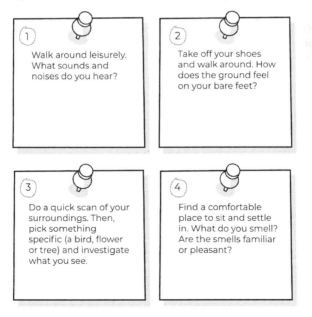

1. Walk around leisurely. What sounds and noises do you hear?

2. Take off your shoes and walk around. How does the ground feel on your bare feet?

3. Do a quick scan of your surroundings. Then, pick something specific (a bird, flower or tree) and investigate what you see.

4. Find a comfortable place to sit and settle in. What do you smell? Are the smells familiar or pleasant?

PAUSE AND REFLECT

- *What types of formal mindfulness practices do you feel most drawn to?*
- *What are some (informal) ways you can bring more mindfulness into your day-to-day life?*
- *How would a regular mindfulness practice benefit your relationship with technology? What about nature?*

CHAPTER 8

Mindset

——————— ♫ ———————

I am always doing what I cannot do yet,
in order to learn how to do it.
—Vincent van Gogh

Cultivating a practice of mindfulness acts like a personal force field that offers protection from the attention economy, and it's a powerful way to bring more intentionality into our lives. Now, we are going to build on that work by exploring our mindsets. This is all about shifting (rewiring) our mindsets to help ensure that the changes we've made have the chance to take root and develop into new habits and lasting effects. This is a key part of the adaptive work for wellness in the digital age.

If you're familiar with the term "mindset," it's probably thanks to Stanford psychologist Carol Dweck. In her book *Mindset: The New Psychology of Success,* Dweck defines mindset as a set of beliefs or attitudes people hold about themselves and their abilities.[96] People with fixed mindsets believe their qualities or abilities are fixed or static, with little room for improvement. People with growth mindsets believe their abilities can be developed and improved with time, dedication, and hard work. For example, someone with a fixed mindset about math would think they are either good or bad at it, and always will be. With a growth mindset, that person would believe that if they consistently applied themselves, their math skills would continue to improve. For obvious reasons, this concept has become popular in many K-12 schools. Ask a tween or teen if they know what "mindset" is and you'll probably get a nod and maybe even a definition. Many teachers are trained on how to nurture growth mindsets in the classroom, and it is often woven into the curriculum and learning outcomes.

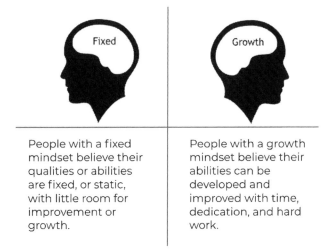

People with a fixed mindset believe their qualities or abilities are fixed, or static, with little room for improvement or growth.	People with a growth mindset believe their abilities can be developed and improved with time, dedication, and hard work.

Why Mindset?

Reframing and developing our mindset is critical when we are trying something new or changing our behaviors and habits. Which, of course, is exactly what the aim of this book is. We're on a journey to adapt to the challenges of living in the digital age by changing our behaviors and finding a different and more balanced way forward.

Back in Chapter 2 we looked at the challenges of living in the digital age through the lens of leadership. A key principle from that chapter was about being able to distinguish between a technical problem and an adaptive challenge. As a reminder, technical problems are often easy to identify, lend themselves to quick and straightforward solutions, and typically can be solved by an expert or authority in the field. Adaptive challenges, on the other hand, don't have a straightforward solution or an expert to consult to find the answer. Adaptive challenges often require changes in values, beliefs, and mindsets, and it is up to the people with the problem to do the work of solving it.

We came to see that the challenges central to this book have both a technical and adaptive component. Solving adaptive challenges requires an individual and family to change and adapt and requires a tolerance for trial and error. Another aspect of an adaptive challenge is that there will inevitably be change, loss, and the need to step out of our comfort zone.

Having the ability to adjust our mindset and look at things from a new perspective is key when dealing with adaptive challenges.

On our journey to wellness in the digital age, things will certainly be challenging at times. There will be highs and lows as we find our way. If we approach things with a fixed mindset, we are almost guaranteed to give up when things get tough and to retreat back to our comfort zone. With a growth mindset, we have the capacity to look at this as a great adventure, a challenge to work through in order to grow and to learn. Of course, this doesn't just apply to your journey of cultivating wellness in the digital age; it applies any time you strive to change and grow, or challenge the status quo and step into the unknown.

Sebastian's Story: Math Mindset vs. Surfing Mindset

Growing up, I always struggled with math. I'm not sure exactly when it happened, probably around second or third grade doing multiplication flashcards, but at some point early on I made up my mind that I was no good at math. From my perspective, it didn't matter what I did or how much I studied, it just didn't compute. I felt like there was something wrong with me, with my brain, and that I was born without the math gene. Because of this belief, my expectations were typically quite low when it came to math through much of my early academic life. Not surprisingly, I developed a very negative relationship with the subject and anything to do with it. I made it into an enemy. My aim was simply to get through it, to graduate, and eventually not have to take math ever again.

Looking back, it's clear that this was a perfect example of developing a fixed mindset early on in my life. When I compare my math mindset to my surfing mindset, it's amazing to see the difference. I grew up surfing from a very young age, and while I did have some natural skills and talents, I always felt like the sky was the limit in what I could do. Any innate talents I had only got me so far. What made the biggest difference was my belief and mindset when it came to surfing. I felt that if I put in the time and effort, I could continue to grow and progress. Any time I ran into a challenge or roadblock with learning a new trick or trying to ride different types of waves, I saw it as a great opportunity to practice longer and to dig deeper in order to figure it out. I had no doubt that with time and practice I would continue to grow and improve. As you can imagine, my trajectory in surfing went up and up, while my trajectory in math dipped and dipped.

It wasn't until after high school that my mindset with math began to change. I was fortunate to have a calculus teacher who helped inspire more of a growth mindset within me. And, while I didn't become a math superstar, I did become much more competent and confident in my ability. I even learned to enjoy math and problem solving. With a growth mindset, it became more like a fun and challenging puzzle rather than something I had to grudgingly fight my way through.

Sure, there are a lot of differences between math and surfing. One I felt like I had to do, and the other I wanted to do. But looking back, my overall performance came down to the drastically different mindsets I had when it came to the two endeavors.

Zones of Comfort

Another way to think about mindset is to imagine three zones of comfort: a comfort zone, learning zone, and panic zone. Each zone is represented in concentric circles, with our comfort zone being in the center.

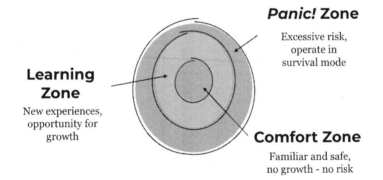

Panic! Zone
Excessive risk, operate in survival mode

Learning Zone
New experiences, opportunity for growth

Comfort Zone
Familiar and safe, no growth - no risk

Our comfort zone is where we feel safe. Things are familiar and predictable to us here. We're relaxed and don't have to think too much. There's no real risk, and subsequently no real opportunity for growth either. This could be relaxing on a nice couch, watching Netflix, and eating your favorite snack. What's in one person's comfort zone (or any zone) is not necessarily the same for someone else. This is on an individual-by-individual basis. For some people, singing karaoke in front of a large audience could absolutely be in their comfort zone. For others, this could be deep in the panic zone.

The next circle out is our learning zone (also called challenge zone). We are now stepping outside of our comfort zone and into new territory. We're not far from the safety of our comfort zone (we can still see it when we look back), but we're doing something different and having a new experience. The risk is not overwhelming, but we're not entirely comfortable either. This is where opportunity for growth and learning exist. If singing karaoke in front of a large crowd feels overwhelming to you, perhaps singing in front of a small group of friends would be in your learning zone.

Beyond the learning zone is the panic zone. Just as it sounds, a panic zone isn't a fun space to be in. Here we have traveled so far outside of our comfort zone, miles beyond our learning zone, that we almost can't function. The experience is one we are woefully unprepared for, and we begin to panic. We become either paralyzed or shift quickly into survival mode because the risk is so overwhelming. Learning and development are practically impossible in this space. The sooner the experience is over, the better—we're just trying to get through it as fast as possible and in one piece!

It's probably clear why we want to be mindful of our panic zone boundary, and how it would be ideal to spend time in our learning zone. It's usually less obvious, though, what the danger of our comfort zone is.

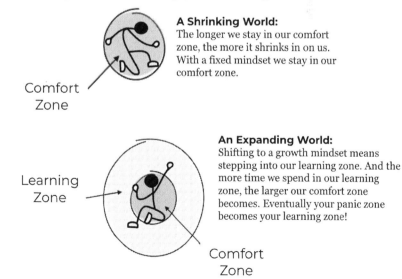

A Shrinking World:
The longer we stay in our comfort zone, the more it shrinks in on us. With a fixed mindset we stay in our comfort zone.

Comfort
Zone

An Expanding World:
Shifting to a growth mindset means stepping into our learning zone. And the more time we spend in our learning zone, the larger our comfort zone becomes. Eventually your panic zone becomes your learning zone!

Learning
Zone

Comfort
Zone

If we get too cozy in our comfort zone and refuse to venture out, the world begins to shrink in around us. Think of your three zones as fluid and evolving. Depending on the experiences you seek (or don't seek), your zones expand or shrink. When you try new things, learn to surf, do karaoke, join a Meetup group, or get dinner with a new friend, your comfort zone expands. When you decline the invitation to dinner for the third time and opt to stay home wrapped in a fuzzy blanket watching Netflix, your comfort zone shrinks.

So, how do our zones of comfort tie into our mindset? With a fixed mindset, we're more likely to stay in our comfort zone. The longer we stay in our comfort zone, the more it shrinks in on us. When we learn to shift to a growth mindset, we spend more time stepping into our learning zone. And, the more time we spend in our learning zone, the larger our comfort zone becomes. Eventually our panic zone becomes our learning zone!

Beginner's Mind

The way Carol Dweck, the psychologist who popularized the term mindset, talks about mindset has been transformative and enlightening to many of us, but it's not the only way to think or talk about mindset. Another key aspect of mindset is developing the beginner's mind. This is similar in ways to a growth mindset and can be a very helpful way to expand our definition of mindset. The concept of the beginner's mind comes from Zen Buddhism, where it is called shoshin. The beginner's mind refers to having an attitude of curiosity and openness when approaching a task or activity, regardless of your skill level or experience, just as a beginner would. This mindset is sometimes referred to as the *child's mind* or the *don't know mind*. While the term "beginner's mind" was made popular by Buddhism, it also exists in many other philosophies and traditions around the world. And, of course, you don't need to be a Buddhist to practice it.

The beginner's mind can be seen as the opposite of the expert's mind. In the expert's mind, mastery has already taken place, and there is nothing left to learn. The renowned Zen teacher Shunryu Suzuki put it beautifully, "In the beginner's mind there are many possibilities, but in the expert's there are few." Of course, this doesn't mean that you can't achieve mastery or become an expert in something with the beginner's mind, but rather that the way to achieve mastery is to approach it with openness and curiosity. From the perspective of the beginner's mind, even an expert or master can continue to learn and grow.

Sebastian's Story: Returning to a Beginner's Mind

As I mentioned earlier in this book, much of my youth was focused on bodyboarding. I was fortunate to grow up near the beach, and I spent as much of my free time as possible at the beach and in the waves. When I started bodyboarding, it was purely for fun. It was all about play. As I got older and more focused on my sport, it began to take on a different feel. In addition to passion and play, there were other factors vying for my attention. I began to compete, and while I certainly wanted to have fun, I also wanted to win. Over the years, more and more of my focus was on winning contests and getting sponsorships. Eventually that included getting the right photos and footage of myself in order to make money as a professional bodyboarder.

While it's great to be able to win and make money, over the years my relationship with bodyboarding changed for the worse. At some point in my career, I lost my passion for the sport. I found myself becoming frustrated and angry if things didn't go my way, I rarely felt satisfied, and something seemed to be missing. If I didn't perform my best in a competition or if the waves weren't good enough, I would easily become distraught. It got to the point where I found myself excited to bodyboard only when there was someone photographing or taking video of me. What had started out as pure passion and a wonderful physical and creative outlet now felt mechanical and empty.

It was around this time in my midtwenties that I began to experience an intense pain in my left hip. I didn't change my routine much at first. I tried to push through it and figured the pain would go away. It only got worse. As the pain grew more intense, I even had to step away from bodyboarding altogether. After trying many different forms of rehabilitation and physical therapy, I eventually underwent surgery. The surgery and the process of recovery was extremely challenging. I was laid up for weeks and out of the water for longer than I had ever been before. Much of the difficulty for me was that a great deal of my identity and self-worth were connected to bodyboarding. *Who would I be if I couldn't bodyboard anymore?* I thought to myself.

While I struggled during that challenging recovery, an interesting thing happened in the aftermath. After surgery, I slowly but surely made my way back to yoga, surfing, and the physical activities I loved. My hip injury and the rehabilitation process turned out to be a wonderful teacher. Prior to surgery, I had taken so much of my physical ability for granted. During my recovery process, even going on a short walk under my own power was a gift.

I experienced a shift in the way I approached physical activities. My surgery and recovery was like hitting a reset button. It was an opportunity to start anew, to see that my physical ability did not dictate my sense of self-worth. I returned to surfing and bodyboarding motivated by what's inside me—my love and enthusiasm for the sport—rather than doing them to impress or prove myself to others, or out of the fear of what I'd lose if I didn't do them. The process has been one of returning to a childlike wonder and joy.

I'm still very interested in progressing and honing my skills, only now there is a renewed sense of freedom, fun, and creativity. I've had a similar experience with my yoga practice. Before surgery, my sense of self-worth was connected to my ability to do advanced postures and my focus was on looking the part of a master yogi. Post-surgery, my practice has been about honoring my body and doing exactly what I am able to do. Like bodyboarding and surfing, I still pursue new knowledge and continue to develop my practice and do so with a different mindset.

Stepping Into Your Learning Zone

Developing a growth mindset and cultivating a beginner's mind are essential for wellness in the digital age. Throughout this process of creating healthy boundaries with technology, reconnecting with nature, and building our capacity for mindfulness, practicing the beginner's mind is invaluable. Let's say, for example, that one of your goals is to replace 30 minutes of screen time with 30 minutes of unplugged nature time at a local park. If you're able to bring a beginner's mind to your 30-minute walk in the park, even if you've been there a hundred times before, you'll find the experience novel and fresh. It helps us to approach activities, school, work, and people with a sense of wonder and curiosity.

Similar to mindfulness, the intellectual understanding of shifting your mindset and stepping into your learning zone isn't very helpful unless you can put it into practice. As we mentioned before, everyone's learning zones are unique. It's important to get in touch with what our individual comfort, learning, and challenge zones are. It's not until we've identified them that we can actively and intentionally move out of our comfort zones and into our learning zones. And the goal is to be spending much more time in our learning zones than we typically are. The following activity will help you begin this process.

Activity: Develop a Growth Mindset

Our comfort zone keeps us in familiar spaces that are free from risk but offer no opportunity for growth. When we step into our learning zone, we are choosing new experiences that allow us to learn, even if it feels uncomfortable or scary.

I will do one thing every week that pushes me into my learning zone.

My comfort zone looks like:
- ☐ Watching TV/Movies
- ☐ _____
- ☐ _____
- ☐ _____
- ☐ _____
- ☐ _____
- ☐ _____

My learning zone looks like:
- ☐ Getting coffee with a new friend

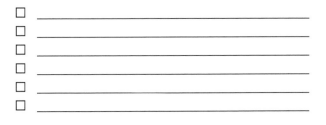

PAUSE AND REFLECT

- *What is one area of your life in which you tend to stay in your comfort zone? What are some ways that you can explore stepping into your learning zone?*
- *What's an area in your life that you tend to approach from an expert's mind (this could be your work, school, hobby, relationship, etc.)? How could you bring more of the beginner's mind to that area? What would that look like?*

CHAPTER 9

Inner Alignment

⌇

Values are like fingerprints.
Nobody's are the same,
but you leave 'em all over everything you do.
—Elvis Presley

We know the pull of the attention economy is powerful, and we've worked on different ways to stay grounded and centered amongst all the digital distractions. We've built our muscle of attention through mindfulness and started to shift our mindsets. From a leadership perspective, this is the adaptive work. Now, it's time to continue that work by strengthening our inner alignment. We like to think of this as a north star: a light to guide us when things get challenging on our journey. To strengthen our inner alignment, we'll clarify and focus on what we want (our internal motivation), take steps to shift from the fear of missing out (FOMO) to the joy of missing out (JOMO), learn how to deal with disappointment, and dive deeper into our personal values.

Internal vs. External Motivation

A big part of wellness comes from being actively engaged in what we are doing. This engagement can come from within or be driven by outside sources. Things like our job, school, friends, and family are examples of inputs that are outside forces or external motivation. When it comes from the inside, or internal motivation, it's driven by our own want and desire. It's not one or the other; rather, we are all motivated by a combination of internal and external factors.

One of the things we focus on with our clients, and key to wellness in the digital age, is how to get in touch with our internal motivation. When we're in touch with our internal motivation, we can stay focused on our goals and values. It also helps us notice when we start heading in the wrong direction and can more easily course correct. Instead of getting pulled into the vortex of the attention economy, we can use internal motivation as our compass or north star, safely and successfully navigating the changing seas of the digital age.

We're not trying to give external motivation a bad rap. There will continue to be external pulls for all of us, like pursuing a job promotion, getting a new car, or winning first place and getting that shiny trophy. If we're totally at the whim of external motivators, though, we'll run into problems. The important thing, and our goal here, is that we make the internal drivers primary and the external motivators secondary, because they affect our well-being differently. The pursuit of internal goals is associated with greater well-being, whereas external goals are associated with lower self-esteem, higher drug use, and a lower quality of romantic and platonic relationships.[97]

Let's look at an example to help bring this to life. Johnny is a high school sophomore and his goal is to get an A in World History. Johnny is much more focused on the external goal (the letter grade) than any internal motivation. He's feeling pressure from his parents to get straight A's and, while he's only a second-year student, he's thinking a lot about his college prospects and future career path. In his mind, he needs this A desperately. It will either make or break him. As a result, his focus is completely on the outcome, and he does whatever it takes to get the A. In class he's attentive but not very interested in the actual content being taught. Instead, he's carefully listening for anything the teacher says about papers, quizzes, exams, and anything that is remotely grade-related. He homes in on the study guides the teacher provides.

His experience of class is one of general anxiety and high stress. When it comes to studying, he aims for rote memory to recall important dates about battles, treaties signed, and other key points of the course. He stresses and crams and pulls all-nighters to prepare for quizzes and tests. At the end of the semester, Johnny achieves his goal and gets an A. However, his experience of taking the course was filled with stress and anxiety. What's more, his grasp of the course content and his retention of the important points was almost nonexistent.

Now, let's look at a different approach. Sally is in the same class as Johnny. She also has the external goal of getting an A in the class.

What's more important to her, though, is her internal goal, the pursuit of learning. She's developed a passion for history, for the stories and power struggles and all the different dynamics at play. She's actively engaged during class, asks lots of questions, and is there to learn and grow. She also pays attention to the papers, quizzes, and tests, but looks at them with a growth mindset—as challenges rather than obstacles. When it comes to studying, she carefully reviews the study guides and dives deeply into the readings in order to learn more. She also comes away from the class with an A, but her experience of the class was completely different from Johnny's. It was one of engagement and challenge rather than anxiety and stress. Not to mention, she's retained a great deal of information that will serve her well moving forward.

From the example, we can see that internal and external goals and motivation are not mutually exclusive. They can work well hand in hand. We can also see from the example how focusing solely on the external goal can become problematic. The gains and satisfaction are short-lived and the experience is often high-stress. Let's take a closer look at what happens when our motivation primarily comes from the outside.

The Hedonic Treadmill

What happens when we are driven by external motivation alone? We end up on what's called the hedonic treadmill. The concept, also known as hedonic adaptation, states that if we're driven only by external motivators, shortly after we reach our goals we'll end up back where we started. No matter how big our achievement or success is, our level of happiness will quickly return to a pre-established baseline and the cycle will begin again.

The treadmill analogy is perfect. When we're chasing external goals, our pursuit of happiness and satisfaction never ends. We'll stay in continuous motion, but never move forward. If we reflect on times in our lives when we've really wanted an external goal, whether that's getting a new car, partner, house, or work promotion, there was probably a fantasy attached to it. By attaining that goal, we fantasize that our self-worth and value will increase and we'll be substantially happier. We'll finally "be set," and our life will be better. But, what really happens? We get the new car, we're ecstatic, and we feel amazing. This new ride is a game changer. But within a relatively short period of time, whether it's a few days, weeks, or months, things start to change. The new toy starts to lose its appeal, we get disappointed with it, or a newer, faster version comes out, and we're back where we started. Then we start to eye a new external goal and we're back on the treadmill.

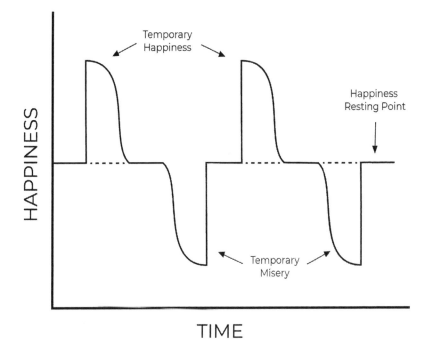

The Hedonic Treadmill

In her book *The How of Happiness*, psychologist Sonja Lyubomirsky makes the case that contrary to what many of us believe, our external circumstances account for a small fraction of our happiness.[98] In fact, according to her research, only about 10 percent of our happiness is determined by our external circumstances—factors like where we were born, our socioeconomic status, etc. What determines the rest of our happiness? What makes up the other 90 percent? According to her book, each person has a different happiness set point, a finding learned when researchers studied identical twins with the same genes. That set point is our genetic predisposition for happiness, and it makes up 50 percent of the equation. The other 40 percent is what we can control and includes things like mindsets, actions, and thoughts, which is why we spend a lot of time talking about internal work in this book.

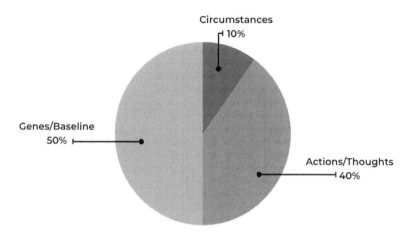

Circumstances
10%

Genes/Baseline
50%

Actions/Thoughts
40%

The How of Happiness Pie Chart

So, how do we escape this cycle and break the spell of the hedonic treadmill? Part of the solution is to get in touch with our internal motivation. While external motivation often has to do with things like money, image, and status, internal motivation often comes from things like self-development, self-awareness, and helping others. When we attain goals that come from an internally directed place, we break the cycle. Instead, we are steadily building up our baseline level of well-being and happiness. In other words, we are improving the aspects of happiness we can control within that 40 percent.

Self-Authorship

Another way to look at internal motivation is that it's self-directed. In leadership terminology we call this self-authorship. It's critical that we feel self-authorized to pursue what we want from within. Instead of pursuing goals that are based on other people's values or interests, we create and follow our own path. We feel self-authorized when we have an opportunity to truly be the authors of our own story. The way we do that, bolster our internal motivation, and build our self-authorship is by getting in touch with what we want. This is at the core and the essence of self-authorship. When it comes to our relationship with technology, we must be clear on what serves us and what gets in the way.

Another reason self-authorship is an important part of wellness in the digital age is that without the "I want," without internal desire and drive, there's an empty space. As we mentioned in the opening of the book, time is our most valuable nonrenewable resource. There are 24 hours in a day, and we can either proactively fill that time or let something or someone else fill the space for us. Either way, that time gets used and the day goes by and another one begins. In other words, if we don't know what we want out of the day, external motivators and unconscious behaviors will take over and fill our time.

Our Values vs. the Attention Economy

As we begin to identify and connect with our internal motivators, we'll also be clarifying our values. This work often happens side by side. We introduced the concept of core values, what drives our personal beliefs and attitudes, at the end of Chapter 2, and we're going to explore them further here. This is all about looking at what we are doing from day to day and whether it's in alignment with our values.

As we know by now, the attention economy does not care about us or what we want. Its sole function is to grab our attention and keep it for as long as possible, regardless of the impact that has on us. If we're not careful, our values will be dictated by advertising dollars and the attention economy. It is as if our values and the attention economy are in a tug of war. When we lose our footing or become disconnected from our values, we're easily pulled over the line and the attention economy wins. Then it becomes the driver in our lives, while our values take a backseat and our internal motivation gets fuzzy.

In his book *Lost Connections*, author Johann Hari dives into how connecting with meaningful values plays a key role in mental health and in fighting against depression.[99] Before talking about the importance of meaningful values, he explores how many of the values our society focuses on are externally driven, superficial, and materialistic. As a way to highlight this, Hari makes an apt comparison between our diets and our values. Just as more and more of us have shifted from eating nutritious food to eating junk food, we have shifted from having meaningful values to having junk values. As Hari wrote in a

Los Angeles Times article in 2018, "Junk food looks like food, but it doesn't meet our underlying nutritional needs. In a similar way, junk values don't meet our underlying psychological needs—to have meaning and connection in our lives. Extrinsic values are KFC for the soul. Yet our culture constantly pushes us to live extrinsically."[100] And, nowhere in our society do these extrinsic junk values get pushed more than in social media and the attention economy.

It may be helpful to look more closely at the values of the attention economy, or rather the values it's promoting to us. Remember, once we're in the attention economy's trance, its values become our values. It happens without us even realizing it. So, what are these values that are being promoted to us? Let's step back and think about this. The attention economy wants us to value our image, money, and social status above all else. It values popularity above substance. In other words, it's based on external and superficial values as opposed to internal values. To borrow Hari's phrase, these are junk values through and through. When these junk values (or materialistic values) become part of our core values, our well-being declines. We're less likely to have experiences that satisfy important psychological needs, and more likely to behave in ways that damage our interpersonal relationships and community connectedness.[101]

Compare the values of the attention economy to the core values that you chose in Chapter 2. Are they in line with your personal values? Probably not. It's extremely helpful to be explicit about that. Remember, the attention economy does not care what your values are. In fact, from its perspective, the less tied you are to your values, the better. This is why it's so important to do the work to connect with values that are meaningful. Doing this is an amazing immunization against the attention economy.

Of course, there is no magic bullet for this, and that's why this is adaptive work. Building our capacity for self-authorship, staying centered on our values and connected to our internal motivation takes time, practice, and perseverance. When we work with our individual coaching clients, we make it very clear that while we are there to help, support, and guide them, it's ultimately up to them to do this work, and no one else can do it for them.

Dealing with Disappointment

We've just spent a good deal of time and energy focusing on the importance of getting in touch with what we want from a self-directed and internal place. It's equally important to talk about what happens when we don't get what we want. That's because getting in touch with what we want does not necessarily mean we'll get what we want. This may seem obvious, but we want to make it explicit. It can be fun, energizing, and exciting to get in touch with what we want, making it tempting to skip over the flip side, but being able to deal with disappointment well is a key component of wellness in the digital age. Remember the difference between technical and adaptive challenges. More specifically, that adaptive work requires change, and with change often comes with a sense of loss. If we're not prepared to deal with disappointment or if we try to avoid or deny the loss, the change will either never happen or it will be unsuccessful.

Each of us reacts to disappointment differently. When you don't get what you want or are having a hard time with a change, what's your go-to response? There are a lot of options available to us. We may throw our version of a temper tantrum. That could be kicking and screaming on the floor or yelling at a stranger on our morning commute in traffic. We may run away, avoid it, or pretend it didn't bother us. We may reach for a comforting food or drink. We may suddenly want to go shopping or have sex. Or—and this option is growing in popularity—we may reach for our phones or turn to digital media.

Our phones have become one of our biggest vices and comforts when we don't get what we want. This is why it's so important to understand the workings of the attention economy. Its power and pull and that of social media is built on the assumption that people don't have the skills to be disappointed well. They're counting on our poor coping skills and the fact that we'll try to self-soothe with our phones by seeking likes, comments, cat videos, or any number of other ways we might get a hit of dopamine—the feel-good chemical that plays a key role in motivating our behaviors—to boost our mood.

What, then, are the inner skills we need to cultivate so that we can be disappointed well? The key to being disappointed well is our ability to get in touch with our emotions. We have to feel those emotions to get to the core of what's happening. Then we can appropriately regulate, heal, and find resolution. The key is to be able to soothe ourselves from within rather than look to the outside world (food, drink, sex, social media) for a solution. Running away or reaching for our phone is an unconscious behavior and an avoidance of feeling what's actually going on beneath the surface. If we have the ability to feel our emotions—to feel sadness, anger, or whatever comes up—and work with disappointment, we then have the ability to soothe ourselves. It puts a bit more space between us and the attention economy. This is bad news from the perspective of the big tech companies—and all the companies that rely on those platforms for advertising space—but great news for us and our health and wellness.

To be clear, we're not saying that all social media or phone use is driven by emotional avoidance or unconscious behavior, just like eating chocolate cake isn't always an avoidance behavior. There is definitely a time and place for chocolate cake and a time and a place for tech and social media. The point is to get in touch with our emotions to raise our level of awareness. Once we have more awareness, we can then ask ourselves: Am I checking social media because I really want to? Or, am I avoiding something deeper? Then we have a choice in the matter, and the dynamic shifts from unconscious to conscious.

Value vs. Experience

Another way of thinking about this is how to be okay when we're not okay, to self-soothe when we're disappointed. One of the best ways to do that is through our ability to discern value from experience. Value, in this sense, refers to our sense of self-worth. Sebastian has been keenly interested in mental health and wellness since he lost his father to suicide as a young boy. For much of his adult life, he's been on a journey of learning and discovery around mental health advocacy and suicide prevention. One of the most powerful lessons he learned through his journey was from Dr. Gregory Dickson, a psychologist and mentor, regarding the concept of value vs. experience. While the frame of this is from a mental health perspective, it is directly related to the inner work of wellness in the digital age.

What does value vs. experience mean exactly? We know that life is full of ups and downs, highs and lows, peaks and valleys, and everything in between. As a human being, it doesn't take too long to realize this. We have a birthday party and get to eat cake. It's amazing! Our favorite toy breaks or gets lost. It's the worst! The highs and lows start early. When we are very young, our experiences (the highs and lows) are directly connected to our value (our sense of self-worth). We're three years old, having a birthday party and eating cake. Our interpretation of that is: this experience is awesome, therefore I'm awesome. When I'm having a great experience, my sense of self-worth is through the roof. On the flip side, let's say we're three years old and are having a nice time playing with our favorite toy when it breaks unexpectedly. This is a bummer. The same thing happens here with the lows. We interpret that experience as: this is the worst, therefore I'm the worst. When we're having a bad experience, our sense of self-worth plummets with that experience. And, that's how it is through much of our early development: our value and experience go hand in hand. Check out the diagram below for a visual representation of this: experience goes up, value goes up; experience goes down, value goes down.

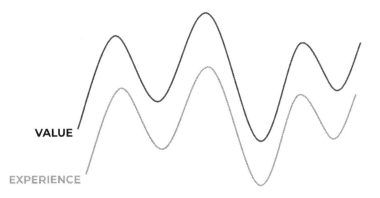

As we get older and we mature and develop, things begin to shift. We begin to separate what happens to us (our experiences) from our sense of self-worth (our value). As we move into adulthood and continue to mature, we may reach a place where our experiences are totally separate from our value. Let's say as an adult we gain a promotion at work. We've been working toward this for a long time. We're ecstatic, and it's an awesome experience! While that's a great experience, we know that we're not a better person because of it. It doesn't raise our value, our level of self-worth. Or, let's say we get into a fender bender in the parking lot. We're angry this happened to us and sad that our new car is scratched and dented. While this is a bad experience, we're now in a place where we know it doesn't make us a bad person; it doesn't lower our level of self-worth. See the diagram that follows. Our value stays flat and unchanged, while our experiences go up and down throughout our lives.

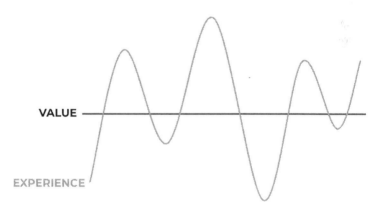

So, how do we work toward separating our value from experience? Developmentally, this typically occurs throughout adolescence as we grow and mature. However, we will all have areas of our lives where our value (self-worth) feels tied to our experience, even into adulthood. We can separate them by reminding ourselves that life's ups and downs are up-and-down experiences, not up-and-down fluctuations in our self-worth or value. Again, the way to get in touch with experience is to get in touch with our emotions. Getting in touch with our emotions helps us stay connected to the experiences we are having moment by moment. What are we feeling at this moment? Mad, sad, glad, or afraid? Those emotions will help us connect to the experience. While we can work toward this place of separating our value from our experience, it's important to understand that it will never be perfect. We all have certain situations and dynamics where our value gets mixed in with our experience. Just as with the practice of mindfulness, our work is to notice and raise our level of awareness to get in touch with the experience directly. Think of this as a practice and a work in progress.

Of course, this whole concept rests on the perspective that we all have personal value. It's our belief that we come into this world with value and we leave it with value. Nothing that we do throughout our lives can affect our value as a human being. With this view, a person who is homeless has the same value as a millionaire who owns a beachfront property. Mother Teresa had the same value as the poor patients she helped and cared for. Our impact on the world, our relationship status, our demographics, our choices will change and shape our experiences, but they do not change our value.

FOMO

Separating our value from experience helps us live well and with intention in the digital age. When we deal with disappointment well, feel and experience our emotions, resist using our phones as an avoidance behavior, and practice separating our value from experience, we're effectively taking the air out of the attention economy's tires. We like to think of it as strengthening our personal force field that protects us from the attention economy. Think about your social media profile (if you have one), whether it's TikTok, Instagram, Facebook, LinkedIn or whatever. If our value and sense of self-worth is tied up in our social media profile, it has a great deal of power and control over us. Not to mention, it can be extremely stressful if we are constantly thinking about maintaining a specific image on our profile.

If our value is connected to our virtual avatar (social media profile), then it's as if whatever happens to our avatar happens to us. If we post a picture and it gets a negative reaction, no reaction, or if people dislike it and make mean comments, it's as if we are being personally insulted and assaulted. As a result, our personal value plummets. On the other hand, if we post something that gets a positive response, abundant likes, and flattering comments, it's as if we are being honored and celebrated, and as a result our personal value skyrockets. You can imagine, or perhaps you know from experience, the stress and distraction that this can cause. Unfortunately, it's the daily reality for many social media users. One of the clearest and most prevalent examples of what causes a negative response (drop in sense of self-worth) on social media is the concept of FOMO.

FOMO (the fear of missing out) isn't a new phenomenon. The fear or anxiety of missing out has been around for ages and has biological roots meant to keep humans connected and vigilant for relevant news and happenings. However, in recent years and largely due to social media and the attention economy, FOMO has evolved and become a daily experience for millions of people. It's so prevalent that it's in the *Oxford Dictionary*, defined as *anxiety that an exciting or interesting event may currently be happening elsewhere, often aroused by posts seen on a social media website.*[102] We consider FOMO one of the secret weapons of the attention economy. It's what keeps many of us coming back to apps and platforms over and over again. FOMO isn't just about what's happening within our friend group on social media; it can be about what's happening on the news, in politics, or in sports. The general anxiety of not being up to date and in the know is what fuels us to check our phones when we have 30 seconds of downtime. It's why many of us are on our phones when we're waiting in line, at a stoplight, on an elevator, or at a coffee shop. It's one of the reasons we stay stuck in unconscious patterns with our devices. Of course, FOMO doesn't just happen when we have downtime. We may be doing something we really enjoy when we get a notification or see something on social media that seems more exciting. FOMO can strike any time and any place.

We have certainly experienced FOMO and know many others who've experienced it as well. In our coaching work, especially with our younger iGen clients (those born between 1995 and 2012), we have been blown away by how often and how intensely many of them deal with FOMO. For some of our clients, the stress is unending and overwhelming. It's an incredible pull, and we have a lot of empathy for young people growing up in this digital age.

It's difficult to be a kid today. When we were growing up (before the introduction of smartphones), FOMO certainly existed, but it was relatively infrequent. We'd show up at school on a Monday and find out that our friends had a party on Saturday night and we weren't invited. It's a terrible feeling, missing out and feeling unwanted, and we had to deal with it from time to time. Today, though, it's like FOMO on steroids. We spoke with a high-school-age client recently who had a similar scenario, but today's hyperconnectivity totally changed her experience. It was a Saturday night, and she found out in real time that her friends were having a party without her. Unlike us, she didn't have a blissful weekend of not knowing until Monday. Through her favorite social media app, Snapchat, she was able to see a play-by-play recap of the gathering through fun and exciting photos as the party went on into the night. What's more, Snapchat has a GPS-enabled feature similar to apps like Uber or Lyft that allows users to track their contacts. With it, she could see all of her friends hanging out at the same address at the same time, without her. Imagine dealing with that level of FOMO! That's just one of many stories we've heard from our younger clients. FOMO is also what encourages many of them to literally sleep with their phones, with sounds and notifications on, so that they don't miss out on any news or gossip overnight.

FOMO to JOMO

FOMO is rough today. It's a major issue, but there is a way out. In recent years there's a concept that has gained some traction which encourages going from FOMO to JOMO. JOMO (the joy of missing out), coined by Anil Dash, a blogger and software company CEO, refers to the gratifying feeling you get when you break away from the (real or virtual) activities of your social group and spend time doing exactly what you want to do most. The idea is that instead of being worried and stressed about all the things we aren't able to know or be a part of, we shift our mindset to focus on the things we can do and want to do.

The shift from FOMO to JOMO can be relatively easy and straightforward. But there are also times when it feels impossible to flip the switch and be joyful about missing out. It can be challenging to suddenly go straight from FOMO to JOMO, and we tend to see it as more of a process and practice that incorporates most of the concepts we've already discussed in this chapter. While it doesn't have to be in this particular order, here are some ways to break the cycle when we're experiencing FOMO:

FEEL YOUR EMOTIONS

When FOMO happens, instead of jumping straight to joy, we may need to slow down and spend a little time feeling the emotions that are coming up. Are we feeling angry, sad, or something else? Avoiding those feelings typically doesn't work out well. Emotions are energy, and if we don't do anything to process them, they will swirl inside us and manifest in any number of ways, like jaw tension, headaches, irritability, distraction, back pain, or high blood pressure. Or, it will turn into some sort of unconscious behavior, like reaching for chocolate cake, a drink, or our phones.

SEPARATE VALUE FROM EXPERIENCE

It's also important to step back and remember to separate our value from our experience. While the experience of FOMO is usually unpleasant, it doesn't actually change or threaten our self-worth. Our self-worth isn't dictated by any experience. What's happening without us is not about us. In other words, FOMO isn't personal.

GET IN TOUCH WITH WHAT YOU WANT

Getting in touch with what we want is all about finding our internal motivation and self-authorship. If we aren't in touch with what we want, FOMO will always sneak up on us and take over. When we're in touch with our internal motivation, we can proactively pursue what we want, which makes it much easier to step into JOMO.

When we let ourselves fully feel our emotions, separate our value (sense of self and self-worth) from the experience, and get in touch with what we want, FOMO disappears. It's also helpful to remind ourselves that we can't do everything or be everywhere. When we do that, we're better able to embrace the joy of missing out, be fully present, engaged, and grateful for whatever we are doing moment by moment. That is what JOMO is all about.

~

By working on our inner alignment, we have built up our personal defenses against the attention economy. We now have the ability to separate our value from what happens on social media (this is equally applicable to the news or any other facet of the attention economy). If our sense of self-worth isn't tied to our social media presence, it will have a lot less control over us and it will be a lot less stressful. We can certainly still use social media in intentional ways that serve us well, but because our virtual profiles are no longer connected to our sense of self-worth, we now have freedom in using them.

Activity: Putting our Values into Action

As a way to further protect us from the attention economy, let's dive deeper into our personal values. Off the top of your head, can you remember what the five values were that you wrote down in Chapter 2? If you're like most of us, you probably remember a few of them, but not all five. And that's interesting, isn't it? Five isn't really that many, and they're supposed to be our core values. These are the values that guide the way we think and behave. Whether you recalled all five or not, it's time to really connect with your values and examine how fully you're embodying them.

Step 1: Rewrite your top five core values

1. _____

2. _____

3. _____

4. _____

5. _____

Step 2: What do your values look like in action? Add a verb to your values to bring them to life.

Example: Curiosity. I approach every day with curiosity.

_____ Rank _____

_____ Rank _____

_____ Rank _____

_____ Rank _____

_____ Rank _____

Step 3: Reread your values in action statements. How fully are they embodied? When you go to sleep at night and reflect on your day, were your values present and alive throughout? Were your behaviors, thoughts, and actions aligned with your values? Take a moment to rank each value from 1 to 10 on how fully embodied it is in your life. A rank of 10 would be *fully embodied* and a rank of 1 would be *not embodied at all.*

PAUSE AND REFLECT

- *Consider the five core values you've identified and ranked. How present and embodied are they in your day-to-day life?*
- *For any value that you feel you aren't embodying (ranked 6 or below), reflect on why that value is not being lived out. What is getting in the way of that value?*
- *What specific shifts (actions/thoughts/behaviors) might you make in order to more fully express your values?*

PART FIVE

RECHARGE

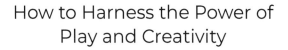

How to Harness the Power of Play and Creativity

We're now at the final part of the ENU Method. The problem was reframed in Part I. We reset our tech and brought more nature into our lives in Part II. In Part III, we broke out of the box and reconnected to our bodies and each other. Then, we dove into the deeper work and rewired our thinking and approach to our daily lives in Part IV. This work is not about just getting to a baseline; it's about getting in touch with what we want and stepping into our potential. We're now ready to explore, adventure, try new things, and engage with life and the world around us in a completely new way. Here we'll look at how to recharge our batteries through the power of play and by bringing more creativity into our lives. By the end of this part, and the end of this book, we will have decluttered our digital lives and reconnected with ourselves, each other, and the world around us. We'll have gone from surviving to thriving in the digital age.

CHAPTER 10

Play

∿

We are never more fully alive,
more completely ourselves,
or more deeply engrossed in anything
than when we are playing.
—Charles Schaefer

It's become the norm in our culture to spend more time and energy focusing on what's not working, the deficits, instead of what is working and our potential for growth. This is reflected in many of our larger systems. Think about our medical model in the United States. The medical model focuses almost entirely on disease and illness and how to remedy diseases. Most doctors and psychologists aren't experts in health and wellness but in particular diseases or pathologies and how to make them better. In essence, the system is set up to keep people alive rather than reaching their full health potential. Modern medicine is amazing and allows us to save people from heart attacks, chronic diseases, mental health crises, and cancer. And, at the same time, there needs to be more focus on preventive and proactive care, on what our health potential could be.

While the medical system as a whole is skewed toward a focus on illness rather than wellness, not all doctors and medical experts take this view. In recent years a lot of growth has taken place in Integrative Medicine and other approaches that are more holistic and focus both on addressing illness and on bolstering wellness. Hopefully, this trend will continue in order to help balance things out.

Unsurprisingly, there is a similar dynamic in the world of psychology and mental health. That system is largely based on the medical model, which focuses on pathology and diagnosis rather than wellness.

Again, not all psychologists and mental health experts fall into this category. Positive psychology, which was introduced in the 1990s by Martin Seligman (but has been around in principle since the early 1900s), is a wonderful example of taking a different and more holistic approach to mental health. Positive psychology is the study of how human beings prosper in the face of adversity.[103]

The goals of positive psychology are to identify and enhance the human strengths and virtues that make life worth living and that allow individuals and communities to thrive.[104] Another view of positive psychology is that it's a scientific approach to studying human thoughts, feelings, and behavior, with a focus on strengths instead of weaknesses, building the good in life instead of repairing the bad, and bringing the lives of average people up to "great" instead of focusing solely on moving those who are struggling up to "normal."[105]

Our approach at Nature Unplugged has been deeply inspired by the field of positive psychology. There is extensive research on the negative impact of technology, social media, and the attention economy. Just as with the medical model, so much of the focus and energy is still on the problem. Our focus, and the focus of this book, has been on what we can do about it. And instead of just trying to repair the bad and get back to baseline, our goal is to help people live well and thrive.

One of the best ways of moving from surviving to thriving in the digital age is by developing a spirit of play. Play is a core aspect of positive psychology and is at the heart of the work we do. When we talk about play, we're not talking about video games or digital games. We're referring to play in nature and outdoors, unplugging whenever possible, and playing with other people. There are incredible benefits, both mental and physical, to bringing more play into our lives. Let's jump in!

The Benefits of Play

There are very real and scientifically proven benefits to play for both children and adults. Play elevates mental performance and heightens levels of attention, creativity, focus, and memory. Play that includes movement and physical activity improves heart and lung function, lowers instances of type 2 diabetes, asthma, high blood pressure, and sleep apnea. It also helps build stronger muscles and bones, improves balance, coordination, flexibility, dexterity, and agility. In terms of social and emotional well-being, play improves social skills, confidence, emotional regulation, and self-esteem, and increases happiness. Developmentally, it also builds critical tactile and sensory motor skills.

- Through imaginative play, children become more creative, perform better at school, and develop a problem-solving approach to learning.[106]
- An IBM Institute survey showed CEOs value employees with creativity, which can be fostered through childhood play.[107]
- Play is strongly linked to stress reduction.[108]
- A 2011 study showed that third graders who had 15 or more minutes of recess a day were better-behaved in school than those who had less.[109]
- According to Dr. Stuart Brown, author of the 2009 book *Play*, play reduces anti-social and criminal behavior, helps couples rekindle their relationships, can facilitate deep connections between strangers and cultivate healing.[110]

Nature Unplugged Play

When we talk about play, we're referring to play activities that fall under one or more of these categories: outdoors, analog, and/or with others. Again, play doesn't have strict rules and we're not trying to limit it here. We're offering these three categories as guiding principles to help you get the most benefit from your play time. Playing outside puts two of our favorite things together and is ripe with positive outcomes. All the goodness and benefits of play and nature are tied together. Keeping things analog (low-tech or no-tech) limits the likelihood of distraction and promotes presence. We feel strongly about play being an unplugged activity.

Otherwise, you could argue that people are playing a lot nowadays. More so than ever before, in fact. There are countless video games and games on our smartphones, computers, and tablets. Many aspects of our social media apps and online experience are gamified to keep us engaged and using them for longer periods of time. Those aren't the types of play we are referring to. While it may be possible to truly play on a device, there are a lot of obstacles and drawbacks that counter the benefits. Play is an opportunity to strengthen our connections with ourselves, others, and the world around us.

Finding a way to insert play into your everyday life is the primary goal. Everyday analog play is good, and we'll feel the benefits of it immediately. What's even better than that is when we can play outside in nature, or play while being totally unplugged. The absolute best way to play—this is both our opinion and based in science—is to play in nature unplugged. It's the best because we get the most from the experience. The benefits are exponentially larger when all three of these things are done together.

The Evolution and Disappearance of Play

When we explored the impact of a sedentary lifestyle and the importance of movement in Chapter 5, we also touched on aspects of play. While movement and play are often intertwined, they are not mutually exclusive. One of the biggest consequences of our increasingly digital lives is that we spend more time indoors and by default spend less time outside playing. One of the things we hear over and over from parents in their 30s and 40s is how fondly they remember their childhood time outside playing, exploring, and roaming the neighborhood or local nature area with friends. They have a genuine deep sadness that their kids don't seem to have the same experience. There's a loss that's felt for their kids, who seem to prefer to spend their free time indoors, alone, engaged with technology and screens. That feeling usually stems from memories of childhood filled with independence, unstructured time, and tech-free play.

The impact of technology and increased screen time is often most noticeable when we look at the effects on kids. That's just one piece of the picture, though. Play has evolved for both kids and adults. The tools we use to play have shifted toward screens, consoles, and smart devices. Instead of playing with physical learning blocks, we turn to a device because "there's an app for that." Instead of playing capture the flag with a group of kids in the neighborhood, kids are connected online and talking to each other from their couches miles apart. Instead of playing an actual game of chess with another human being, adults are playing against computers on their phones.

With so much to occupy our time and attention inside, we're spending less time outside playing and exploring. Additionally, many areas don't have the same access to green and open spaces that they once did, limiting the physical spaces available to play in. The U.S. Forest Service reports that an estimated 6,000 acres of open spaces are converted for other uses every day.[111] This is largely due to development of urban and suburban areas, and often results in the loss of forests, grasslands, and other natural areas.

OBSTACLES OF PLAY

Alongside diminishing green and open outdoor spaces, there are a wide variety of other obstacles that can keep us from living our play potential. Some of the most common roadblocks that get in the way are safety concerns, too much structure, and not enough boredom. These barriers are not age specific. They come up for kids, teenagers, young professionals, parents, and older adults alike.

IS IT SAFE?

One constant task that life gives us every day is identifying, acknowledging, and assessing the risk of our behaviors and our environment. Whether it's at the front of our minds or lurking in our subconscious, we're continuously processing information and trying to sort out what's a real risk and what's perceived or exaggerated. You might ask yourself whether it's safe to meet a few new friends in the park for a hike or a pickup game of soccer. Or, is it okay to let my kids go outside for a few hours unsupervised to goof off, explore, and play around the neighborhood?

While there's a shift in perceived safety—57% of registered voters in the U.S. believed crime had gotten worse since 2008—the reality is that violent crime (rape, robbery, assault) in the U.S. has seen a 50–70% drop from 1993 to 2019 according to the Federal Bureau of Investigation (FBI) and the Bureau of Justice Statistics (BJS).[112] Of course, playing outside isn't risk free, and safety varies from city to city. There are real dangers in the world that we all need to be mindful of, and only you can determine what risks you find acceptable. The point here is to understand that sometimes the danger (and risk) we feel is due to the increasing visibility (not prevalence) of violence and crime today. Knowing the real risk lifts the weight of fear and concern a bit and allows you to enjoy each day more.

TOO MUCH STRUCTURE, NOT ENOUGH BOREDOM

Most kids and adults are also increasingly overscheduled, leading to less boredom and opportunities to incorporate play. And finally, the nail in the coffin is a cultural belief that play is frivolous. Play is often seen as the antithesis of efficiency and responsibility. At younger and younger ages we are encouraging more time on academic pursuits and less time on play and fun. This carries over and intensifies in our adult lives.

Writer and blogger Amanda Rock defines unstructured play as "a category of play in which children engage in open-ended play that has no specific learning objective."[113] Unlike structured play, unstructured play is not instructor-led, so parents, teachers, and other adults do not give directions. It also does not have a particular strategy behind it. Much has been written in recent years about the benefits of unstructured play. In a 2016 article in *The Atlantic* called "In Defense of Play," author Alison Gopnik does a wonderful job of detailing the benefits of play for children (and adults) and explains why unstructured, random play is so important. Gopnik writes, "The gift of play is the way it teaches us how to deal with the unexpected."[114]

As a parent or teacher, you may feel pulled to intervene, give instructions, soothe, or correct misunderstandings. Perhaps you feel pressure to entertain kids and young adults, but it's important to step back and let them entertain themselves. Boredom comes first, self-sufficiency comes second. Adults experience the same resistance to unstructured play that kids do. We tend to overplan or get bored and leave the minute there's a lull in activity. Tight schedules, shorter attention spans, and the nagging feeling that we're supposed to be getting things done prevents us from experiencing downtime. Without the space and time for it, unstructured play can't exist for adults or children. We need to allow kids and ourselves room to roam, to embrace what is commonly referred to now as "free range" living or parenting.

The beauty of play is that it can happen anywhere at any time. It's not prescribed, and the parameters can flex and expand. You can play games with existing rules or make some up. Recently, we had a backyard party where a group of our friends barbequed, listened to music, and played a few lawn games like cornhole, spikeball, and ping-pong. What sticks out the most, though, was a spontaneous juggling game that we played for multiple hours with about eight people joining in. It included a volleyball that we juggled like a soccer ball and a mop bucket that we aimed the ball at every time a song ended. We called it bucket ball, and it was the highlight of the night.

Sebastian's Story: Never Leave the Playground

One of our favorite places to visit is a nearby county park in the northern suburbs of San Diego. It's called San Dieguito Park, and it's a magical place. A section of the park is manicured and "orderly," with open grass fields and play structures. And a large part of the park has protected the indigenous coastal sage scrub vegetation, with a nice trail system that winds through it.

I've been visiting this park regularly for the past fifteen years or so. The space has been a refuge for me and a destination to go to recharge. It's also been a wonderful place to be creative and reflective. I typically meander through the park, varying my route a bit with each visit. At some point I pass by the play areas, and it's here that I've observed a scene that's become more and more common. I'll often see a handful of kiddos running around in the sand, climbing, playing, or exploring the structures. And I see a handful of parents, sitting or standing (mostly sitting), glued to their phones.

It makes sense that while the kids are occupied, it is a good time to catch up on emails, the news, or whatever is pressing. But it's also a missed opportunity to move and to engage playfully with our kids. I have yet to see a parent at this particular playground running around in the sand, climbing, playing, or exploring the structures along with the little ones. I understand that it may seem a little strange, even frowned upon in some settings, for adults to be playing like that in public with their kids. But not only is it a missed opportunity for connection, it's a missed opportunity for adults to let go of their to-do lists, agendas, and emails, and engage in something just for the joy of it. Remember, activities like climbing and crawling, jumping and swinging, are wonderful for us both in terms of movement and in terms of incorporating more play and fun into our day.

If you're looking for encouragement and inspiration in the realm of adult play, we highly recommend a quick Google search for a man named Stephen Jepson. If you visit his website, http://neverleavethe-playground.com/, you'll find an adult who really loves to play. At the time of this writing, Stephen is 80, but what you'll notice soon after exploring his website or watching his videos is that there's nothing old about him. Stephen fills his days with play, curiosity, and all sorts of strange and interesting games, many of which he has made up. His mission is to encourage people of all ages to adopt this mindset of play to promote good health and to have fun while doing it. He's a living example of how movement and play benefits us both physically and mentally. And, he's proof that we can do the same.

Playful Ideas

As a reminder, when we talk about play, we're thinking about how we can play in nature and outdoors, unplugging and going analog whenever possible, and playing with other people. Play doesn't need to incorporate all three of these things at the same time, but the more you can work them in, the better you'll feel afterwards. Here are some ideas to get you started.

SCAVENGER HUNTS

One of the best ways to create a sense of adventure and exploration on any nature outing is with a scavenger hunt. You can buy it or create your own. Work as a team, go at it solo, or make it a competition. There are even scavenger hunts that are specific to local and national parks, though they can be just as much fun when done in your backyard or around the neighborhood!

ANALOG GAME NIGHTS

Make a standing date with family or friends for a game night. It works best if the games are analog, meaning no or low-tech. Games with a little competition are a great way to build relationships. Choose a classic like charades or Scattergories, or learn a new game together. Some of our favorites are Bananagrams, Codenames, Utter Nonsense, and a simple but highly entertaining card game called Taco Cat Goat Cheese Pizza.

THE PARK WITHOUT A PLAN

Find time on your calendar in the next couple of weeks for a park outing. Other than coordinating the date and time, keep the plans as loose as possible. Bring a variety of balls, perhaps a lawn game, definitely a deck of cards and maybe even a wordsearch. Blankets and snacks are also advised. Other than that, let the fun emerge organically with your friends or family.

ADULT PLAYDATES

For a more structured experience, schedule a few adult playdates. Get some friends together and choose an activity that is playful in nature. Go bowling, try a new escape room, play paintball or laser tag, or grab a spikeball set and find some sand or grass to play on. Spending time with friends doesn't always have to be going out for dinner or drinks. Don't be shy in actively planning your next playdate.

NATURE PLAY

There's so much to play with outdoors. There are trees to climb, plenty of places to hide (and seek), and a world of possibilities if we let our imaginations run wild. A fun way to experience nature and play is to create a natural game board. The simplest version is to find four twigs and create a tic-tac-toe board. Then you need to find two sets of five matching pieces (five pine cones and five leaves, for example), and you're ready to play!

Activity: Reclaiming Play and Free Time

NEVER LEAVE THE PLAYGROUND

I will find _____ (minutes/hours) for play every day. By play, I'm committing to a variety of activities that include:

- ☐ Scavenger hunts
- ☐ Analog games and puzzles

- ☐ Climbing trees
- ☐ Ping-pong
- ☐ Capture the flag
- ☐ Hide-and-seek
- ☐ _____
- ☐ _____
- ☐ _____
- ☐ _____

UNSTRUCTURED FREE TIME

I will ensure that every weekday has at least _____ minutes/hours of free, unscheduled time.

I will ensure that every weekend day has at least _____ minutes/ hours of free, unscheduled time.

PAUSE AND REFLECT

- *When was the last time you felt a sense of wonder or awe? Is there a way to bring more wonder into your life? How might you do that?*
- *What types of nature unplugged play are you most drawn to?*
- *What are the biggest obstacles for you when it comes to incorporating more play into your day? Given those obstacles, what are ways you can mitigate or overcome them?*

CHAPTER 11

Creativity

༄

Imagination is more important than knowledge.
—Albert Einstein

If you give a four-year-old child a new toy or device without any instructions, the child will figure out how to use it much faster than you will; a 2014 study out of UC Berkeley found this to be overwhelmingly true.[115] Why is that? Because children are infinitely more curious and tend to have an open mind. In other words, they have fewer assumptions and biases. When faced with a creative problem-solving task, kids will try all sorts of unusual or impractical ideas to find a solution. Essentially, their thinking has fewer limits.

As we grow older, we tend to become more practical and slowly shed our curiosity and imagination. We trade in our creative outlets and pursuits for more responsible endeavors. When we ask adults who attend our workshops, "When was the last time you made or created something?" many of them have a difficult time coming up with examples. However, creativity does not fit in a box, and almost all of them have recently made or created something (despite what they think). It's not just fine art or music. People make and create things all the time—new recipes, handmade gifts and greeting cards, DIY home projects—but very few believe they are creative. And when we don't think we're creative, or think it's frivolous, we shy away from it and our creative world shrinks. All of the potential benefits and opportunities for growth slip away.

Sonya's Story: Naturescapes

Over the summer, we typically run ENU Adventures that are small group half-day outings for kids, teens, and families aimed at experiencing nature unplugged. Typically held in local parks, lagoons, beaches, and nature preserves, our adventures are a great opportunity to get outside, explore, and take breaks from our screens. We hike, explore, play, talk about leadership, and work in some opportunities for creativity.

One morning, I was out with a group of 11-to-13-year-olds, two girls and one boy. We were just wrapping up our nature adventure, and a lot of their earlier energy had faded and I began to see some heavy eyelids. I threw out my blanket, made out of old jeans that had been sewed together in patches, and we all sat at the edges facing each other. It had been overcast all morning and the ground was still a bit dewy. There weren't that many people in the park, and we had a nice little corner of it to ourselves as we sat nestled under some large eucalyptus trees. "Okay," I said, "We're going to make some naturescapes!" The younger boy immediately groaned and slumped his shoulders, clearly not excited about the idea. The two girls seemed neutral and were being polite, but it was obvious they were ready to get on with the rest of their day.

Undeterred, I told them to get out their notebooks and pens and that it was time to draw. A brief flash of anxiety crossed their faces. I quickly assured them that what they were about to create would not be hung up in a museum, and that by the end of the activity, we'd have four bizarre masterpieces. They relaxed a little, but their hesitancy still lingered. I charged on, "Step one. Choose a spot that you can see right now and focus on that. Draw the ground, the trees, and the sky. Focus on creating the larger landscape." Their pens slowly started moving. Then they started working a little more quickly as their landscape came to life. At the end of four minutes, it was actually hard to get them to put their pens down. "Pass your notebook to the right," I said. They all looked at me a little confused, but then reluctantly handed off their freshly penned landscapes to the person to their right.

Next, we added in a few animals to the scene and passed on the drawings again. Then, some water features and weather. Finally, we added a few people. When our notebooks finished the rotation and made it back to the original artist, the piece of work was ridiculous and delightful. We all were allowed to add a few final touches, and then placed the notebooks in the middle to view our masterpieces together.

As we oohed and ahhed and laughed about the final pictures—the 11-year-old boy added rampaging dragons and crocodiles to each picture—the energy of the group had completely changed. There was a lightness about us and smiles across the board. Everyone was fully awake and engaged. The transformation was incredible, as it always is by the end of this activity.

Creative Possibilities

No one has zero creativity. It can come in the form of artistic expression, but it might also be finding a solution to a problem that no one had thought of yet. It's the ability to come up with original, useful, imaginative or innovative ideas. Basically, creativity is a huge umbrella that lots of things fall under, and we all tap into it daily. Creativity is an outlet, a stress reducer, a mental exercise and practice, and an opportunity for growth and personal development. It's those things and more, but what it's not is frivolous or a waste of time. In fact, creative expression and work can stimulate the neurological system and enhance health and well-being.

HOW CREATIVITY IMPACTS THE BRAIN

When we talk and think about our brains, we often oversimplify things into left-brain/right-brain functioning, with our left brain managing logic and analysis while our right brain takes care of creation and innovation. While still oversimplified, Grant Hilary Brenner, MD, offers a different way to think of creativity and the brain by focusing on how "the big three" brain networks operate together as a team.[116] Many researchers believe that Albert Einstein's genius—academically and creatively—was from the continuous development of the different hemispheres and networks in his brain. His brilliance came from developing and training each part of his brain to work together as a high-performing team.

The big three networks are the default mode network, the executive control network, and the salience network. The default mode network is basically the brain's resting or idle state. The executive control network is the brain manager; it manages emotion, directs attention, and makes decisions and choices. The salience network is the information filter, determining what makes it through and is noticed versus what gets unprocessed and goes unnoticed. In reviewing the current research, Dr. Brenner notes that creativity requires all three of those brain networks to work in coordination and can be developed and improved. Creativity improves our brain function. It boosts our cognitive functioning, sharpens our senses, and is a positive cycle that inspires innovation.

EMOTIONAL AND PHYSICAL WELL-BEING

Scientifically speaking, happiness is felt when dopamine, the feel-good chemical, is released in our brains. When we successfully create something, such as a painting or a poem, learn to play a new song, or refinish an old piece of furniture, dopamine is released in our bodies. The more you like the final product and the more time you put into it, the larger the dopamine release is. Regardless of whether you notice your boost in happiness, that chemical response will influence and encourage you to create again.

Creative tasks often require focus and repetitive motions, offering benefits similar to meditation and opening up opportunities to achieve flow, both of which reduce anxiety, depression, and stress, and produce a general calming effect. Girija Kaimal, assistant professor of creative arts therapies at Drexel University, co-authored the study "Reduction of Cortisol Levels and Participants' Responses Following Art Making."[117] A total of 39 adults who ranged in age from 18 to 59 were asked to participate in a 45-minute task where they could choose to color, play with clay, or create art collages. This study found and supported the finding that expressing ourselves through art can significantly lower the cortisol (the stress hormone) in our bodies. What we found most interesting about the study was that many participants stated they had little to no opportunity for art-making as adults.

Additionally, there are numerous studies that show how creative outlets can help people process trauma. In a comprehensive article, "The Connection Between Art, Healing, and Public Health," Heather L. Stuckey and Jeremy Nobel explain that writing, painting, and drawing can be a tool for people to express themselves and make sense of their experiences when words are too difficult or painful to use.[118]

Less well known are the physical benefits of creativity. According to Stuckey and Nobel, expressive writing has been linked to reductions in physician visits and better immune system function.[119] Additionally, listening to music stimulates the brain in ways that regulate hormonal processes and the body's inflammatory response. Another study by Graham et al. found that writing and expressing angry feelings helped with chronic pain management. Over a period of nine weeks, participants experienced improved pain control and a decline in pain severity.[120]

Art and creativity also offer outlets for personal exploration and growth. There are an endless variety of tools and mediums available to us—fine arts, crafts and hobbies, repurposing old items, home projects and renovations—all equal in their opportunity to create and find joy and satisfaction. Art gives us opportunities for self-expression, a child-like freedom and playfulness, a chance to experiment, make mistakes, and improve. Consistent creative adventures and pursuits build resilience, self-awareness, and self-confidence.

NATURE AND CREATIVITY

Not only does nature relax the prefrontal cortex and give the brain a break, it also activates what's called the imagination network. Remember, as our prefrontal cortex quiets down, it allows the rest of our brain space to work in coordination. When we don't have to focus on anything intensely or specifically, our brain's default mode kicks in and our minds can wander. The imagination network is essential to creativity because it lets ideas flow, both memories and visions of the future. It lets us reflect and create meaning. It awakens our sense of awe.

A 2012 study from Tel Aviv University found that awe led to increased creativity by opening the mind or prompting expansive thinking.[121] Often in nature we are confronted with the vastness of oceans, forests, mountains, and deserts. It can make us feel small in comparison, and that feeling leads to awe. Stunning and peaceful naturescapes also lead to soft fascination, similar to a meditative state or fully relaxed mind, which is also known to activate our imagination networks. Nature inspires curiosity, encourages us to relax our bodies and minds, inspires creativity, and helps us overcome creative roadblocks.

There are countless stories of people having moments of profound creativity while in nature. Even leaders in the tech industry have had some of their greatest insights outdoors. A great example of this is the experience of Marc Benioff, the founder and CEO of Salesforce.

com, one of the leading enterprise cloud computing companies in the world.[122] In 1996, Benioff, who was feeling burnt out and unfulfilled with his job at Oracle, decided to take a sabbatical to travel and think more deeply about his career and the tech industry as a whole. After spending some time in India, Benioff landed in Hawaii, taking time to enjoy the natural beauty and warm waters. It was while exploring the beaches in Hawaii, and specifically while swimming with dolphins, that he had an epiphany that inspired him to leave his job at Oracle and create Salesforce.

Sonya's Story: Unplugged Creativity

It had been a long day and I was exhausted. A heat wave was making its way through the area and it was blistering hot outside, which is rare for coastal San Diego. After six hours at a local park hiking around with clients, I was a sweaty mess and excited to take a cold shower for some temporary relief. I couldn't wait to eat dinner, curl up on the couch and watch some TV. Sebastian and I had settled in and were watching one of our favorite TV shows. Each episode ended with a cliff-hanger, and we gladly rolled into the next one without much thought. About halfway through the third episode of the evening, I started feeling anxious and unsettled. I paused the show and was about to check in with Sebastian when he said, "We need to move the TV out of the living room." I totally agreed. Our living room is our main living space, and we spend the majority of our time there. We couldn't seem to help ourselves from getting sucked in, but I wasn't sure I was ready to say goodbye to our TV yet, so I said, "Let's sleep on it."

The next morning, when I woke up, removing the TV was the first thing that popped into my head and it was the first thing I did (after coffee, obviously). We put a picture up where the TV had been and moved the TV into the garage, then got on with our day. When the evening rolled around, we were a little awkward as we tried to fill the void TV shows had filled. Boy, was it tempting to fill the space with other forms of technology. But we managed, and the next day was less awkward. We started asking each other more questions, our reading time soared, and I even got Sebastian to play a few board games with me. The most interesting thing was that my creativity skyrocketed. The void that TV left offered space for my mind to wander, and my imagination and curiosity kicked in. I started writing notes to myself with new ideas. I started singing and making up funny songs to sing to Sebastian while we were making dinner or cleaning up. My crafts came alive again, and so did my art. It had been years since I had last painted or drawn anything more than a doodle. I rediscovered so many creative outlets and felt energized in a way that I hadn't for a long time. All it took was moving our TV fifteen feet away and into a different room.

Reconnect to Your Creativity

Whether you identify as creative or feel like the creative gene skipped you, there's probably room for more creativity in your life. Notice and make note of obstacles to getting started. Maybe it's too much screen time. Perhaps it's a lack of supplies. It can also feel uncomfortable or scary to try something new, or maybe you're just unsure of how to get started. It's extremely important to understand that art and creation are not some divine gift bestowed upon you at birth. It's like anything else. It requires practice, mistakes, resilience, and persistence. There is no right or wrong; there's just creating or not creating. Start small, manage the obstacles you can, disconnect from your devices and screens, and give it a try. If you don't know where to start, here are some ways to push outside of your comfort zone and into your creative zone.

A NOTEBOOK IN NATURE

Grab a notebook and pencil and sit outside on your balcony, patio, a neighborhood bench, in a park, or your backyard—whatever is available to you will work fine. Set a timer for 30–45 minutes and let yourself write, doodle, or draw anything you want. Give yourself total freedom to create.

MAKESHIFT MUSIC

One of the best things about music is that you need very little to make it. You can sing, whistle, clap your hands, or stomp your feet. A bucket can become a drum, two sticks can be knocked together to keep a tempo, and a glass and a spoon can make a beautiful chime. Of course, there are traditional instruments too. Whatever you have, and whatever inspires you, have an outdoor jam session, solo or with a friend.

PAINT EXPLORATION

Abstract painting is a fun place to start, regardless of your skill level. Explore what's around you. Zoom in on a leaf or a flower. Notice the colors around you and just begin putting them to paper. Try to use the brush strokes to create movement on your paper. Throw blotches of paint down, or let your brush drip colors in different places. If you want, add complexity with different mediums (pen, pencil, pastels, paper).

COLLAGE AND MIXED MEDIA

Sometimes a piece of blank paper can be intimidating. We get it. When that happens, it can be helpful and inspiring to pull out some colored paper or magazines to find a color or image that sparks an idea. Cut it out and paste it down. That's where you start, and then see where you go from there. You can draw, paint, or write in the free spaces. When you feel any hesitation, let go and remember there are no rules—it's your piece of art!

PAPIER-MÂCHÉ

It can be messy, but it's always fun. All you need is an idea, some paper (newspaper, notebook paper, construction paper, etc.), and some watered-down adhesive (usually water and glue). You can make a mask, an animal or figurine, or maybe even a bowl or hat. The sky's the limit here. After a short drying period, you have a 100% unique creation.

DAILY HAIKUS

Commit to a 30-day haiku challenge. You might scribble a quick haiku down on some days and spend an hour thoughtfully examining a flower for inspiration other days. Every day, though, you'll write a three-line poem. A traditional Japanese haiku has seventeen syllables and is written with a 5/7/5 syllable count.

FUNCTIONAL CREATIONS

Creativity and function can coexist, from handmade jewelry to baking to home improvement projects and everything in between. Take a minute to connect with something you've been meaning to get to or try out. Get the tools you need—clasps, beads and string, a recipe and the ingredients, or a sander and some paint—and get to it!

DECORATIONS AND DECOR

It's not just what's framed and hung on your wall; works of art can take many forms. Ditch the canvas and paint a mural, make a personalized banner for an upcoming birthday, or create your own unique holiday decorations. What's missing in your house, bedroom, or apartment right now? How can you create it yourself this month?

JOIN THE KIDS' TABLE!

If you have friends with children, or are a parent, teacher, aunt, uncle, or grandparent, find a way to draw, paint, sculpt, build, or bake with kids. The messier the better. The sillier the better. One of our favorite things to do with kids (and adults) of all ages is to bring Play-Doh—or as we like to call it, nature putty—outside with us! Everyone can sculpt the things they see around them. Use fallen leaves, sticks, and nuts to create imaginary creatures, or create a full nature scene as a group.

Activity: Reconnect to Your Creativity

Remember that art and creation are not some divine gift bestowed upon you at birth. It's like anything and everything else. It requires practice, mistakes, resilience, and persistence. There is no right or wrong; there's just creating or not creating.

I will do the following creative activities:

Every day...
- ☐ Write
- ☐ Doodle or draw
- ☐ Play music
- ☐ _____
- ☐ _____
- ☐ _____

Once a week...
- ☐ Write a song or poem
- ☐ Paint
- ☐ _____
- ☐ _____
- ☐ _____

Once a month...
- ☐ Do a home improvement project
- ☐ Make a handmade gift
- ☐ _____
- ☐ _____
- ☐ _____

PAUSE AND REFLECT
- *How has your definition of creativity changed?*
- *What are three ways you can bring more creative energy into your life?*
- *What are some ways you can use nature to encourage creativity?*

CONCLUSION

Engaged Living

—————————— ∿ ——————————

To live is the rarest thing on earth.
Most people exist, that is all.
—Oscar Wilde

Lancaster, Pennsylvania, is home to the largest Amish population in the United States, just under an hour's drive from where I (Sonya) grew up. Whenever we found ourselves heading east, noticing the landscape shift to rolling hills and windmills, my sister and I would keep our eyes peeled for buggies. I remember being fascinated whenever we spotted members of the Amish community traveling on the road by horse. It seemed like we had traveled back in time. What would make an entire community choose a horse and buggy over a car? It just didn't make any sense to me.

That wasn't the only interaction my family had with the Amish; we'd also see them frequently at our local farmers market. My mom and dad always made a point to stop by their stands when we'd pop in. They made the best pastries and bread, apparently. More than that, I remember how they dressed. I thought they were dressed up as Pilgrims, that they were wearing costumes to help with sales. Clearly I didn't understand their way of life, but I was extremely curious about it. When Sebastian told me about a documentary series he had come across called *Living with the Amish*, I was eager to check it out and learn more about a community I grew up so close to and yet was such a mystery to me.[123]

Living with the Amish

The documentary series, *Living with the Amish*, follows a group of eight British teens as they leave behind their modern urban worlds full

185

of technology and convenience and temporarily live with Amish families in Ohio. For context, the Amish live interesting and intentional lives. There are many rules and regulations that govern their community. They commonly travel by horse and buggy instead of by car. They often have strict guidelines regarding technology, choosing not to tap into the electrical grid, use self-propelled farm machinery, or own devices like televisions, computers, or radios. To be clear, technology is not banned outright in Amish communities. Instead, new technology is closely examined and scrutinized. Before allowing tech into their community, the Amish weigh the potential benefits against the potential harm or distraction and whether it supports their values.[124] While much of their lifestyle and culture seems antiquated and even archaic, one thing is certain: their rules and customs promote a high degree of presence, intention, engagement, and sense of connection throughout their community

When the group of British teens arrived to meet their Amish hosts, a young married couple in Middlefield, Ohio, they felt as if they had landed on another planet. The teens wondered why anybody would want to live like the Amish do. Almost immediately, the teens had to give up their devices. All of their smartphones, iPads, computers, and other gadgets were kindly but firmly collected by the Amish couple. Of course, that was just the tip of the iceberg. The teens then switched their wardrobes for traditional Amish dress, which included sewing and making parts of their own clothing. Once the teens were outfitted, there was a welcome dinner and celebration for the guests, which was short-lived before the chores and work began.

The women spent most of their time cleaning the house, repairing clothes, and preparing the meals for the day. The men were out tending to the farm, livestock, and property, and chopping wood for the furnace for heat and hot water. This group of teens was diverse, but they had all grown up in the city. Back in London, they were savvy and modern young adults. When it came to the Amish way of life, though, they were inexperienced in basic skills and had little to contribute. In the beginning, they had no idea how to exist or operate. Once the teens were taught how to do the work—whether to shovel, wash up, or sew a pair of pants—an incredible shift took place. They went from being apathetic and resistant to engaged, empowered, and even excited to work.

Within a few days you could see the boost in their confidence, and it carried over to other aspects of their lives. They started to hold themselves differently, their posture shifted, and their communication changed. They stopped missing their phones, social media, and old way of life and began to be fully present in what they were doing and engaged with the work that needed to be done. It's a powerful example of the changes that can take place when people (no matter what age) shift from passively going through life to actively engaging in it.

Engaged Living

Engaged living is the end game. It's what we're talking about when we say our work is to help people thrive in the digital age. Engaged living is about being fully in the moment and proactively playing a part in what is happening all around. It brings together all of the different themes and concepts we've talked about in this book. When we're engaged with life, we're able to appreciate what we have and actively pursue our goals. It's about choosing to hold tech boundaries in order to create more space in our lives, choosing to spend more time in nature, choosing to move our bodies, choosing to practice mindfulness and develop a growth mindset, choosing to connect to our core values, choosing to play, create, adventure, and explore. Engaged living isn't about what you do, the activities themselves; it's more about how you do them. It could mean doing the same job you've been doing for fifteen years but doing it with intention, with care, and taking time to really connect with your coworkers and customers.

As a result of the attention economy and the challenges of living in the digital age, many of us are on the verge of apathy, which is the opposite of engaged living. Apathy is what happens when we are not in touch with what we want, and it creates a sense of nothingness, like living in a vacuum. In large part, this happens because of all the convenience, ease, and comfort that comes from modern technology. It produces a surplus of time. Having more free time sounds like a good thing, and it is in many ways. There are lots of pros to it, but the con is that we're constantly confronted with the choice of how to spend our time and where to focus our energy. If we're not in touch with what we want, we'll end up doing whatever is easiest and takes the least amount of thought and energy. This is passive living. We become disengaged, and life starts to speed by us. We spend our time playing video games, constantly checking our email, or scrolling through social media feeds and the news. Not because it's what we want to do, but simply because it's the path of least resistance.

There are many of us who are on the flip side of that same coin. Our day is jam-packed, with every minute scheduled and an endless to-do list. It's a little less intuitive, but this is usually an avoidance of engaged living, too. Busyness does not equal engagement. If we are disconnected from our values and what we want, we say yes to everything and everyone. We try to do it all because we aren't clear on what's important and what's not. It takes practice and persistence to live an engaged life. It's a muscle we have the capacity to build. To do this, we need to be willing to take risks and push outside of our comfort zones. Time is a gift, and it's up to us to spend it in ways that bring us joy, happiness, health, passion, inspiration, fun, and connection. That's engaged living.

Moving Forward

We have made our way through the ENU Method. By now, we are well informed and understand the pull of the attention economy and the challenges of living in the digital age. Even though we dream of a quick fix, we know that a healthy relationship with technology requires deeper work. We've hit the reset button and have boundaries in place that minimize digital distractions and promote a nature-rich life. We've adopted a new mantra of sit less, move more. In addition to reconnecting with our bodies, we've pushed ourselves to engage with each other and connect to our communities. As for the inner work, we've built and strengthened our force field against the attention economy. We've done this through cultivating a practice of mindfulness, developing a growth mindset, and reinforcing our inner alignment through getting in touch with what we want and our core values. And last but not least, we've found time and space in our day for play and creativity. We're not just going through the motions anymore, simply existing. We're moving through our day with engagement, purpose, and intention. Though we will certainly face obstacles and disappointment, we are primed for a life of wellness in the digital age.

When we first introduced the ENU Method, we presented each part in a sequential order. The process is very much like making our way up to the peak of a mountain. We started at base camp with "Reframe," and over the course of our journey worked our way up to the peak, to "Recharge." Each step built on the next and prepared us for what was to come. While the steps are presented in the optimal order for learning and integration, the reality is that our journey toward wellness in the digital age is an ongoing process rather than a specific destination. It's more like a circle or continuum rather than a path to a peak. Each part of the ENU Method is fluid and ever changing.

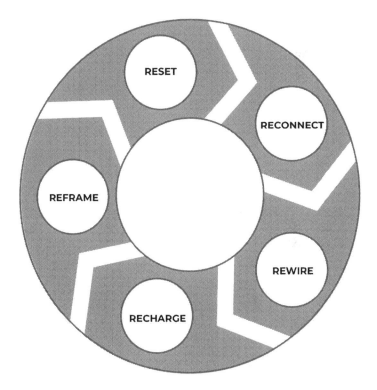

As our lives and technology evolve and our family and relationship dynamics change, we will have to change with it. The tech boundaries that worked well for us when we were young will probably need to change as we get older. Having a full understanding of the method and each part of the process allows us to revisit, adjust, and focus on specifics as needed.

189

Philosophy and Contract for Wellness in the Digital Age

When it comes to bringing this work into our lives moving forward, one of the best ways to do this is to create a Philosophy and Contract for Wellness in the Digital Age. As we have mentioned, having the knowledge and understanding of what to do is critical. But what's more important is putting it into practice. Your philosophy is a short (one- or two-paragraph) statement that helps guide your path forward. It helps give you the 30,000-foot view and the bigger-picture vision. Your contract, on the other hand, offers more concrete and actionable ways to put your philosophy to work in your day-to-day life. The two combined are powerful tools that will support you in your pursuit of wellness in the digital age. In the appendix you'll find templates and instructions to build these out and help put what we've learned into action. When you're feeling uncertain about your pursuit of wellness in the digital age, return to this philosophy and contract to help guide your decisions so that they align with your values.

~

In the beginning of this book we mentioned the movie *Wall-E*, a story about the dystopian future where humans have used all of Earth's resources and are fully dependent on technology. Our aim at Nature Unplugged, and with this book, is to keep *Wall-E* a fiction. Of course, we don't need to flip our lives upside down and live like the Amish do to avoid the future envisioned in *Wall-E*. We do, however, need to keep our eyes open and make thoughtful and intentional decisions with the technology in our lives and how we're choosing to spend our time. This, of course, brings us full circle to how we opened the book. Knowing that time is our most valuable nonrenewable resource, how do you want to spend yours?

CONCLUSION

APPENDIX I:
Philosophy for Wellness in the Digital Age

The purpose of this activity is to help you build your personal, family, or team philosophy for wellness in the digital age. Thinking back on the work we've done throughout this book—the activities and reflective questions—use the following building-block prompts to distill and clarify your final philosophy.

TECHNOLOGY USE: *Technology offers benefits and distractions. How do you want to be using technology moving forward?*

CONNECTION WITH NATURE: *Connecting with nature is key to our well-being. What does connection with nature look like to you?*

TIME AND VALUES: *Time is limited, and our values guide our actions and shape who we are. With that in mind, how can your values inform how you spend your time?*

Now you have the building blocks for your philosophy for wellness in the digital age. When you're feeling uncertain about life or a new opportunity, the philosophy you're creating will help guide your decisions so that they align with your values. This statement will inspire confidence in each step of your journey.

Next, you'll put your short answers together and draft your philosophy. Be sure to put your sentences in the present active tense. Here's an example from the time and values prompt.

Original statement: *I want to remember to live each day to the fullest.*

Changed to the present active: *I live each day to the fullest.*

Example Philosophy: The following example is from one of our clients who wrote her philosophy with the help of her family.

We use technology with purpose and intention in ways that serve us rather than deplete us. We strive to be present with each other as a family and make space for quality time by having dinner together, playing games, picnics and other activities. We go on fun family adventures on a monthly basis. We achieve balance by taking time to get outside and move regularly and by taking short unplugged breaks throughout our day. We send our tech to bed by 9 p.m. each evening, and this helps us to create tech-free time on a nightly basis. This is an opportunity to read a physical book, stretch, relax, meditate, pray, or whatever serves us best to get a good night's sleep. We will counter the impact of the attention economy by participating in attention-building activities (yoga, mindfulness, time in nature, etc.) on a daily basis. We will be there to help remind each other that family is a priority over technology.

Once you're happy with your draft, write your philosophy on the template on the following page. Or if you'd prefer, visit www.natureunplugged.com to find a free printable version of this template to use, and display the final copy in your home!

DRAFT: _____

_____

_____

_____

_____

_____

_____

_____

_____

_____

_____

_____

_____

_____

_____

_____

_____

_____

_____

_____

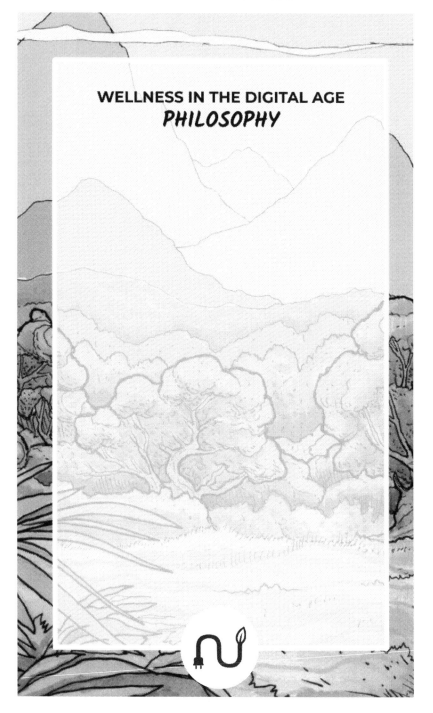

WELLNESS IN THE DIGITAL AGE
PHILOSOPHY

APPENDIX II:
Experience Nature Unplugged (ENU) Contract

Your philosophy will broadly guide your path forward, and now it's time to get more specific by creating a contract. A contract offers more concrete and actionable ways to put your philosophy to work in your day-to-day life. The two combined (your philosophy and contract) are powerful tools that will support you in your pursuit of wellness in the digital age.

We've created a template for your contract that includes a number of items we strongly recommend. The sections from the contract are aligned with the flow of the book and the ENU Method. If you'd like, you are certainly welcome to add any additional contract items to the end of this document or cross out items that don't work for you. Read and complete the following contract individually, as a family, or as a team. For a free printable version of this contract, visit our website at www.natureunplugged.com.

RESET: TECHNOLOGY

CREATE A DIGITAL CURFEW

Your "Digital Curfew" is the time you'll put your devices—phone, tablet, laptop, TV, and video games—to bed for the night, and the time you'll start using them again in the morning. We'd recommend 1-2 hours before you go to sleep and after you wake up.

I will create the following digital curfew:

Each morning I will not use technology/devices before: _____ (a.m.)

Each evening I will put my devices to sleep by: _____ (p.m.)

NO TECH IN THE BEDROOM

Devices in the bedroom tend to stimulate you, either with bright light, sound, or engaging content. None of those are great for preserving your ability to get a good night's sleep.

I will keep the following devices out of the bedroom:
- ☐ Cell Phone
- ☐ TV
- ☐ Laptop
- ☐ Tablet
- ☐ Computer
- ☐ Video Games
- ☐ _____
- ☐ _____
- ☐ _____
- ☐ _____

FIND A HOME FOR YOUR PHONE

Create a "Home for your Phone," a place where your phone lives when you're not intentionally using it. It's where your phone goes and stays until you're ready to intentionally use it again.

The home for my phone will be located:
- ☐ In a basket by the front door
- ☐ At a charging station in the living room
- ☐ _____

SCHEDULE UNPLUGGED TIME

We recommend scheduling at least 60 minutes of unplugged time every day (outside of your digital curfew time). This unplugged time could be all at once during an unplugged walk, workout, craft, favorite hobby, or reading time.

I will unplug every day for _____ minutes. My intention is to take:
- ☐ One long break of at least 60 minutes
- ☐ Two 30-minute breaks
- ☐ A few smaller breaks of 5–15 minutes each
- ☐ _____
- ☐ _____

CREATING ROUTINE WITH BOOKENDING

We highly recommend bookending your day with a tech-free morning routine and an unplugged evening routine. This could include things like stretching, meditation, exercise, reading a physical book, doing a crossword puzzle, etc. Find what works for you and explore working it into your schedule.

Each morning I will do the following before starting the rest of my day:
- ☐ Exercise/Walk
- ☐ Stretch
- ☐ Journal
- ☐ Read
- ☐ Meditate/Pray
- ☐ Take Time in Nature
- ☐ _____
- ☐ _____
- ☐ _____
- ☐ _____
- ☐ _____

Each evening I will do the following before going to bed:
- ☐ Stretch
- ☐ Journal
- ☐ Read
- ☐ Meditate/Pray
- ☐ Walk
- ☐ _____
- ☐ _____
- ☐ _____
- ☐ _____
- ☐ _____

TECH-FREE ZONES & TECH-SPECIFIC SPACES

Designating spaces that are tech-free (in addition to the bedroom) or tech-specific helps create and manage expectations of where you will and won't be using technology in your home.

Phones, computers, tablets, and other smart technology are not allowed in the:

- [ ] Dining room table
- [ ] Backyard
- [ ] Bathroom
- [ ] Kitchen
- [ ] _____
- [ ] _____
- [ ] _____
- [ ] _____
- [ ] _____

Phones, computers, tablets, and other smart technology are allowed in the:

- [ ] Computer station
- [ ] Office/Home office
- [ ] Desk
- [ ] Phone charging station
- [ ] Entertainment room
- [ ] _____
- [ ] _____
- [ ] _____
- [ ] _____

CREATE WINDOWS OF TIME FOR COMMUNICATION

Just because we can call, text, and email friends, family, and colleagues 24/7 doesn't mean it's a good practice. Set specific times to call, text, and email for better time management and productivity. It's also helpful for staying present in the office, classroom, or when you're with family and friends.

I agree to the following:

- [ ] To call colleagues/clients/classmates during the hours of
_____

- [ ] To call friends and family during the hours of
_____

- [ ] To text colleagues/clients/classmates during the hours of
_____

- [ ] To text friends and family during the hours of

☐ To email colleagues/clients/classmates during the hours of
_____

☐ To email friends and family during the hours of
_____

☐ _____

☐ _____

SET SCREEN TIME LIMITS

Almost all smartphones, tablets, and computers have settings that allow you to set screen time limits. You can set general usage time limits or time limits for specific apps and games. This is a great way to hold yourself accountable, raise your screen time awareness, and encourage intentional technology use.

I will use screen time limits on our/for:
- ☐ Cell Phones
- ☐ Computers
- ☐ Laptops
- ☐ Tablets
- ☐ _____
- ☐ _____
- ☐ Specific websites:

_____

_____

_____

- ☐ Social media platforms:

_____

_____

_____

MANAGING NOTIFICATIONS

What do you need to know right away and what can wait? Most notifications are not urgent and don't require your immediate attention, but when that ding comes through, it's hard to resist the urge to look.

I will turn off all notifications on my cell phone except:

□ _____
□ _____
□ _____
□ _____
□ _____

I will use the "Do Not Disturb" feature for the hours of _____ (a.m./ p.m.) to _____ (a.m./p.m.) and while:
- □ Spending quality time with family and friends
- □ During meals
- □ In meetings or appointments
- □ _____
- □ _____

I will manage the applications on my devices by:
- □ Clearing my home screen and placing all apps in one folder
- □ Using the search feature on my phone to open the specific app I'm looking for
- □ _____
- □ _____
- □ _____

RESET: NATURE

TAKE NATURE BREAKS (5 MINUTES)

Whatever your typical day looks like right now, most of us have the opportunity to take a quick break every few hours. A chance to step away and step outside. The point of a break is to restore, relax, and reenergize. Instead of fitting one more thing in, checking the news, email, or social media feeds, use that time to take a nature break. Remember, just 5 minutes can boost your mood and positive emotions.

I will fit 5-minute nature breaks into my schedule as much as possible:
- □ Before work/school
- □ During lunch
- □ After dinner
- □ In between classes or meetings

☐ When I get home from work/school

☐ _____

☐ _____

☐ _____

☐ _____

☐ _____

To help me achieve this, I will:

☐ Put nature breaks on my calendar

☐ Find a partner to hold me accountable

☐ _____

☐ _____

☐ _____

☐ _____

GET YOUR DNA (15 MINUTES)

When we talk about DNA, we're talking about getting our Daily Nature Adventure. Find 15 minutes every day to get your daily dose of nature while mixing in some novelty and adventure. As we learned, spending at least 15 minutes a day in nature changes our physiology by lowering our cortisol levels (stress), blood pressure, and heart rate.

I will find 15 minutes every day for my Daily Nature Adventure. The best times for my DNA are:

☐ Right when I wake up

☐ Just before breakfast

☐ During lunch

☐ After dinner

☐ In between classes or meetings

☐ Right after work/school

☐ Just before bed

☐ On the weekends

☐ _____

☐ _____

☐ _____

☐ _____

Activities in support of DNA:

- ☐ Taking a stroll in a local park or nature space
- ☐ Urban birding
- ☐ Dipping my toes in the ocean, lake, river, or creek.
- ☐ Walking barefoot outside
- ☐ Jumping in puddles or climbing trees
- ☐ Working out outdoors (nature gyms)
- ☐ _____
- ☐ _____

To help me achieve this, I will:
- ☐ Put DNA on my calendar
- ☐ Find a partner to hold me accountable
  (Name/s: _____)
- ☐ Expand my adventure circle to include
  (Name/s: _____)
- ☐ _____
- ☐ _____

GO ON ENU ADVENTURES

Once a week, find a couple of hours on your calendar to Experience Nature Unplugged (ENU) and go on a mini adventure. These adventures should be just different enough from your daily routine that they create excitement and energy around the experience. They can be relatively short, easy, local, and cheap without skimping on the fun. Adventures can take many forms and be refreshing, rewarding, relaxing, or challenging.

I will go on weekly ENU Adventures that include:
- ☐ Picnics in the park
- ☐ Watching the sunset from a new viewpoint
- ☐ Backyard camping
- ☐ Sunrise hikes
- ☐ Neighborhood birding adventures
- ☐ Ocean dips
- ☐ Visiting new parks, reserves, or trails
- ☐ _____
- ☐ _____

☐ _____
☐ _____
☐ _____

Nature places I have access to and will explore are:
☐ Local parks (like: _____)
☐ My backyard and front yard
☐ Nearby nature spaces (like: _____)
☐ Beaches (like:_____)
☐ _____
☐ _____
☐ _____
☐ _____
☐ _____

To help me achieve this, I will:
☐ Put ENU Adventures on my calendar
☐ Find a partner to hold me accountable
   (Name/s: _____)
☐ Expand my adventure circle to include
   (Name/s: _____)
☐ Embrace the weather and go outside in the rain, wind, cold, heat, or snow
☐ _____
☐ _____
☐ _____

COMMIT TO THREE DAYS EVERY THREE MONTHS

Finding and committing to three days of nature unplugged every three months can be a daunting task, but the benefits of the three-day effect are huge and worthwhile.

Every three months, I will find three days to unplug and immerse in nature by:
☐ Taking local camping trips
☐ Planning nature-based vacations
☐ Turning off Wi-Fi and camping in the backyard

☐ Visiting local parks or nature spaces three days in a row

☐ _____

☐ _____

☐ _____

BRING THE INSIDE OUTSIDE

Are you living most of your life indoors? If so, what activities can be shifted outside? We tend to get into routines that keep us inside, though many of our daily activities are easy (and sometimes more fun!) to do outside.

I will do the following activities outside:
Every day...

☐ Reading

☐ Playing games or music

☐ Exercising

☐ Eating meals

☐ Being social

☐ _____

☐ _____

Once a week...

☐ Reading

☐ Playing games or music

☐ Exercising

☐ Eating meals

☐ Being social

☐ _____

☐ _____

Once a month...

☐ Reading

☐ Playing games or music

☐ Exercising

☐ Eating meals

☐ Being social

☐ _____

☐ _____

BRING THE OUTSIDE INSIDE
In addition to getting outside more, there are a few natural elements you can incorporate in your home to bring nature to you.

I will invite nature into my home by incorporating the following:
- ☐ An indoor herb garden
- ☐ House plants
- ☐ Air plants
- ☐ Natural scents/Oil diffuser
- ☐ Wooden furniture
- ☐ Natural decor
- ☐ _____
- ☐ _____
- ☐ _____
- ☐ _____
- ☐ _____

RECONNECT

RECONNECTING TO OTHERS
As social beings, we need human connection. It's essential for our physical health and mental well-being. In a time when we are prone to self-isolation, we have to consciously seek interaction and connection with friends, family, and members of our community.

I will prioritize social connection over comfort and convenience by:
- ☐ Joining a Meetup group
- ☐ Signing up for an adult rec league
- ☐ Starting or joining a book club
- ☐ Talking to a stranger every day
- ☐ Skipping the self-checkout line
- ☐ Hugging friends and family
- ☐ Cuddling with my partner
- ☐ Getting a pet
- ☐ _____

☐ _____

☐ _____

AIM FOR A HIGHER QUALITY OF COMMUNICATION

The highest quality of communication you can get is an undistracted, in-person, face-to-face, old-fashioned conversation because it yields the most information. However, having an in-person, face-to-face, undistracted conversation is not always possible. The key is to aim for the highest form of communication that you can, given your resources and circumstances.

Whenever possible, I will prioritize the quality of my communication over comfort and convenience by:

☐ Putting my phone away when I'm with friends or family
☐ Calling instead of texting when I have the time
☐ Sharing important news in person
☐ Reaching out directly instead of checking a social media page for updates
☐ _____
☐ _____
☐ _____
☐ _____

RECONNECTING TO OUR BODIES

Any movement is better than no movement. But the absolute best thing we can do to counter the effects of sitting in front of screens all day is to find ways to move our bodies, be outside in nature, and unplug.

I commit to getting _____ minutes/hours of movement every day.

To help me achieve this, I will:

☐ Put movement on my calendar
☐ Use nature as my gym
☐ Go on a walk without my phone
☐ Get out of the box with big stretches and crawling
☐ Embrace the weather (instead of using it as an excuse)
☐ Take breaks from wearable tech

☐ _____
☐ _____
☐ _____
☐ _____
☐ _____

REWIRE

PRACTICE MINDFULNESS

Building our capacity for attention and intention is like anything else. It takes time and practice, similar to going to the gym to get in better shape, build muscle, or become stronger. Find a mindfulness practice that resonates with you and create a standing practice.

I will incorporate the following formal mindfulness practice/s:
☐ Yoga (_____/week)
☐ Breathing Meditation (_____/week)
☐ Mindful Walking (_____/week)
☐ Mindful eating (_____/week)
☐ Tai chi (_____/week)
☐ Body scan (_____/week)
☐ _____
☐ _____
☐ _____

I will incorporate the following informal mindfulness practice/s while:
☐ Washing dishes (_____/week)
☐ Walking in nature (_____/week)
☐ Standing in line (_____/week)
☐ Driving (_____/week)
☐ Talking to a friend (_____/week)
☐ Doing the laundry (_____/week)
☐ Showering (_____/week)
☐ _____
☐ _____
☐ _____

DEVELOP A GROWTH MINDSET

Our comfort zone keeps us in familiar spaces that are free from risk but offer no opportunity for growth. When we step into our learning zone, we are choosing new experiences that allow us to learn, even if it feels uncomfortable or scary.

I will do one thing every week that pushes me into my learning zone.

My comfort zone looks like:
- [ ] Watching TV/Movies
- [ ] _____
- [ ] _____
- [ ] _____
- [ ] _____

My learning zone looks like:
- [ ] Getting coffee with a new friend
- [ ] _____
- [ ] _____
- [ ] _____
- [ ] _____

WORKING TOWARD INNER ALIGNMENT

Getting in touch with what we want, from an internal place, takes time, patience, and persistence. To do this, we need to practice saying no and learn to deal with disappointment.

By keeping my values in mind, I will say NO to things that are not important to me or that take me away from the things I care about and want to prioritize.

My values and priorities are...
- [ ] _____
- [ ] _____
- [ ] _____
- [ ] _____
- [ ] _____

I will say no to...

- ☐ _____
- ☐ _____
- ☐ _____
- ☐ _____
- ☐ _____
- ☐ _____

When I'm disappointed or upset by something that has happened, I will seek the following outlets to process and feel my emotions:

- ☐ Talk to a trusted friend or family member
- ☐ Go for a walk outside
- ☐ Release some energy through exercise or working out
- ☐ _____
- ☐ _____
- ☐ _____
- ☐ _____

RECHARGE

PROTECT YOUR SLEEP

Getting enough sleep helps you have better energy throughout the day and boosts your creativity and cognitive functioning. When we sleep well and long enough, we're generally happier and less irritable. The National Sleep Foundation recommends that teenagers should sleep between 8-10 hours a night and young adults and adults between 7-9 hours.

I commit to getting _____ hours of sleep every night.

While this may vary, my aim is to be asleep from _____ to _____ .

NEVER LEAVE THE PLAYGROUND

Play is important to our happiness, health, wellness, and creativity. Regardless of how old you are, finding time and space for play in your life is critical to your well-being.

I will find _____ (minutes/hours) for play every day. By play, I'm committing to a variety of activities that include:
- ☐ Scavenger hunts
- ☐ Analog games and puzzles
- ☐ Climbing trees
- ☐ Ping-pong
- ☐ Capture the flag
- ☐ Hide-and-seek
- ☐ _____
- ☐ _____
- ☐ _____

UNSTRUCTURED FREE TIME

In addition to play, it's important not to overschedule yourself. Downtime lets us rest and recharge. Without it, our brains and bodies get overworked.

I will ensure that every weekday has at least _____ minutes/hours of free, unscheduled time.

I will ensure that every weekend day has at least _____ minutes/hours of free, unscheduled time.

RECONNECT TO YOUR CREATIVITY

Remember that art and creation are not some divine gift bestowed upon you at birth. It's like anything and everything else. It requires practice, mistakes, resilience, and persistence. There is no right or wrong; there's just creating or not creating.

I will do the following creative activities:

Every day...
- ☐ Write
- ☐ Doodle or draw
- ☐ Play music
- ☐ _____
- ☐ _____

Once a week...
- ☐ Write a song or poem
- ☐ Paint
- ☐ _____
- ☐ _____

Once a month...
- ☐ Do a home improvement project
- ☐ Make a handmade gift
- ☐ _____
- ☐ _____

SIGNATURES:

I/We understand and agree to the terms of this "Wellness in the Digital Age" contract.

Printed Name	Signature	Date

Printed Name	Signature	Date

Printed Name	Signature	Date

Printed Name	Signature	Date

Printed Name	Signature	Date

APPENDIX III:
Formal Mindfulness Practices

Below are brief descriptions and instructions for four formal mindfulness practices to explore: a breathing meditation, a body scan, an eating meditation, and a walking meditation. This is by no means an exhaustive list of options. The idea is to give you a feel for some of the different practices as a foundation to build on. The instructions provided can be used for your own practice or to guide a group. For additional mindfulness resources and pactices, visit our website at www.natureunplugged.com.

BREATHING MEDITATION

Description: Mindful breathing can be practiced to bring attention to the present moment, as a practice of gratitude, to bring in more quiet and space, to notice your thoughts and emotions, and to enhance self or group awareness. Breathing meditations can be practiced first thing in the morning, before going to bed, before eating a meal or snack, while at a beautiful lookout, or whenever it works best for you.

Instructions: Below is a step-by-step guide to this practice.
- Find a comfortable place to sit. Lying on your back is also an option.
- If you're sitting, sit upright but not rigidly.
- Close your eyes. If you're not comfortable closing your eyes, soften your gaze.
- Begin by bringing awareness to your body.
- Take a moment to scan your body.
- Notice any sensations that you feel: warmth, coolness, tingling, tension, etc.
- If you notice any areas of tension or tightness, see if you can soften or relax those areas.

[Option to have participants bring awareness to surrounding nature sounds, or smells, or sensations of coolness or heat from the wind or sun.

The point here is to wake up the senses and bring awareness to the present moment. Spend a minute or so bringing awareness to body sensations.]

- Now bring your attention to your breathing.
- Breathe in and out through your nose if that's available to you (of course, if you're congested, breathe through your mouth).
- Follow each inhale and each exhale.
- There is no need to control your breath. Just notice and follow your breath.
- There are many ways to feel your breath: through the nose and throat, or the rise and fall of your chest, or the rise and fall of your belly.
- Bring your attention to your belly; focus on the rise and fall of your belly. Rising or expanding on each inhale, and falling or contracting on each exhale.
- Focus on the feeling of your breathing as best you can.
- When you notice that your mind has wandered away from your breath, gently bring your attention back to your belly and the feeling of your breath.
- This may happen many times during your practice. The key is to notice your mind wandering and then bring your attention back to your breath, again and again.

[When your allotted time is complete: Option to gently ring a bell or verbally bring the group back together]

- When you're ready, you can open your eyes.

BODY SCAN

Description: Body scans can be practiced as a way to check in with our bodies and notice areas of tension, aches, discomfort, or pain. It can help calm and center a group, be used for self-care, or as a practice of gratitude. You will need a place to sit or lie down comfortably. This can be practiced at a variety of times throughout the day and is ideal during relaxation or downtime. For example, a body scan can be used after a yoga practice or before going to bed.

Instructions: Below is a step-by-step guide to this practice.

- To begin, find a position to sit, recline, or lie down in (whatever is most comfortable to you, as you'll stay in this position the entire time).
- Allow your eyes to close.
- Bring your awareness to your breathing.
- Follow each inhale and exhale.
- Feel the rise and fall of your chest and belly, not trying to control the breathing in any way, simply noticing your breathing as it is.
- Now bring your attention down to your feet and toes.
- Notice what's happening in your feet and any sensations you may feel—coolness, tingling, warmth. If there's any tension there, see if you can relax or loosen it.
- Bring your awareness up to your lower legs and knees, again, noticing any sensations as you move your awareness up your body.

[Depending on how much time you have, you can get more or less detailed. For example, during a longer practice you can focus on each individual toe and make it more specific and in-depth. For a shorter practice, do a more general body scan.]

- Bring your attention to your thighs and upper legs.
- Feel your hips and notice any sensations there.
- Allow your belly and chest to be fully relaxed so that you can breathe easily.
- Let your back settle into the floor.
- Bring your awareness up through your shoulders, relaxing down through your arms, forearms, hands, fingers.
- Move your attention back up through your arms to your neck, head, and face.
- Relax the muscles of your face. Relax your jaw, soften the muscles around your eyes, relax through your hair.
- Now, see if you can bring your awareness to your entire body all at once.
- Try to feel what's happening in your body, noticing any and all sensations, resting in your awareness.
  [longer pause]

217

- When you're ready, open your eyes. You can begin to bring some movement back and wiggle your fingers and toes, wrists and ankles.

[When your allotted time is complete: Option to gently ring a bell or verbally bring the group back together to acknowledge the end of the practice.]

EATING MEDITATION

Description: Mindful eating can be practiced as a way to bring gratitude and presence to your meal and each other and to bring quiet and space to your eating experience. This can be practiced at a variety of times throughout the day, during a snack or as part of a meal. This practice requires at least fifteen minutes and should not be rushed. Allow enough time to slowly eat your snack or meal, minimizing any possible distractions.

Instructions: Below is a step-by-step guide to this practice.
- Hold the food in your hand and bring your full attention to it. Look at it as if you've never seen it before. Examine the different colors, ridges, intricacies of the food. Ask the group to share what they notice.
- Think about everything (all the resources) that went into getting this piece of food into your hands here and now.
- What resources were needed to grow this food? [water, earth/soil, sunlight, pollinators, seed/plant/tree/animal, etc.]
- What about human resources? [farmers/field workers]
- What went into processing this food? [machinery/people]
- How did this food get to us? [transportation, fuel, drivers, cashiers]
- Can you think of any other resources/people involved in getting this food to us?

[After exploring the origin of your food, bring your attention back to examining the food.]

- How does the food feel in your hand? Is it smooth, hard, light, heavy, etc.? Ask the group to share some examples of what they feel.

- Bring the food to your nose and explore how it smells. What aromas/smells do you notice? When you smell the food, do you notice anything happening with your stomach or mouth? [Ask the group what they notice.]
- Now bring the food up to your mouth, but not in your mouth yet. Notice any sensations that come with the anticipation of eating.
- Place the food in your mouth WITHOUT chewing and explore it there for at least ten seconds. Notice the flavor and texture.

[We typically eat with little attention given to the experience of eating; take your time in this final step of the practice.]

- Now, chew the food slowly and notice the different sensations and tastes.
- As you continue to chew without swallowing, notice if the taste or texture changes.
- When you are ready, you can swallow the food. Make an effort to remain aware of the sensations in your mouth, throat, and stomach as you finish eating.

WALKING MEDITATION

Description: Walking meditations offer an opportunity to engage all of your senses and increase your presence. This practice heightens your awareness of your natural surroundings and body through movement. This can be practiced during a hike or short walk. One nice thing about this practice is that you can incorporate it into a functional walk (getting from point A to B). Or, if you'd prefer, walk solely for the meditative practice. It's especially nice when there is beautiful scenery that can be used to increase your appreciation for the surrounding environment.

Instructions: Below is a step-by-step guide to this practice.

The instructions are pretty straightforward. Once the practice begins, it is done in silence. You are going to walk with the intention of being present with yourself and your surroundings. To begin, bring awareness to your body and your breathing. As you start your walk, there are a few options you could focus on:

FOOTSTEPS:
- Bring awareness to each step that you take.
- Feel each step as your foot makes contact with the earth.
- You can imagine that the earth is a big animal and you are massaging its back with each step that you take.
- Or, if it's helpful, you can count steps up to ten, and then start again back at one.

SENSES: In addition to feeling your footsteps, tune in to your senses:
- Feel the coolness of the breeze and warmth from the sun.
- Pay attention to the sounds around you.
- Notice the different sights and views around you. Focus on something small like a rock or flower, or take in the views in the distance.
- Pay attention to what you smell.

ACKNOWLEDGMENTS

We are deeply grateful for all the people who have helped bring this book to life. To the family, friends, teachers, and mentors who helped guide us along the way, some of whom we've mentioned here and many we haven't. To Patti Fox, one of our dearest friends and first clients, for your ceaseless belief, love, and support along the way. We miss you every day, and your life and work continues to inspire us.

To our clients, who have been our constant companions on this journey. We're continuously impressed by your courage and eagerness to step into this process. We learn as much from you as you do from us. To Dr. Mark Kalina and Dr. Gregory Dickson. Your wisdom, expertise, and perspective have informed and transformed our work. To Monica Stapleton, thank you for your unwavering support and valuable insights.

To our professors, mentors, and colleagues at San Diego State University, The University of California at Los Angeles, and The University of San Diego: Diana Richardson, Dr. Christine Wilson, Dr. Robert Naples, Dr. Terri Monroe, Dr. Lorri Sulpizio, Dr. Ana Estrada, Dr. Zachary Green, Dr. René Molenkamp, Kelly Sloan, Mark Ceder, Linda Dews, Dr. Ann Garland, Dr. Erika Cameron, Dr. Wendell Callahan, and Dr. Stefano Olmeti. Thank you for your dedication, encouragement, and guidance.

To our amazing editors, thank you for your clarity and support. To Liz Bandy, for helping us pull all our wild ideas together and keeping us on point. To Frank Steele, for your amazing editing, insights, and help in refining this book.

To our families, for all their love and support along this wild ride. We couldn't have done this without you. And, to honor our fathers, Vernon and Ahmed, for being the greatest teachers we could have ever asked for.

Finally, we'd like to acknowledge and give gratitude to modern technology and our natural world. Technology, thanks for Wi-Fi, the interwebs, and all of the amazing conveniences and solutions you provide. To our natural world, thank you for being a place of refuge, source of creativity, inspiration, and wonder throughout our lives. Nature, you rock!

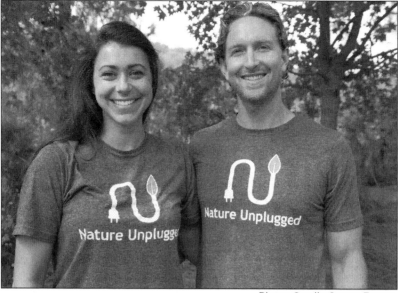

ABOUT THE AUTHORS

Sebastian Slovin and Sonya Mohamed founded Nature Unplugged in 2012 with the mission of inspiring wellness in the digital age. They have developed a unique curriculum to help individuals, families, educators, and organizations break free from the clutches of technology overuse, reconnect with nature, and engage with life and work in a whole new way. For more information, visit their website at https://www.natureunplugged.com.

Since Sebastian can remember, nature has been a central part of his life. He was fortunate to grow up in the beach community of La Jolla, California, and spent his childhood mixing it up in the ocean. As a young boy, he lost his father to suicide, which would deeply inspire his path in life. As a young adult, he had the opportunity to travel extensively and experience many of the world's great surf spots as a professional bodyboarder. Through his travels, Sebastian developed a deep love and appreciation for our natural world and at the same time was drawn to the practice of yoga and mindfulness. His love for yoga led him to study at Prana Yoga Center in La Jolla, California, and his passion for nature led him to pursue a BA in Environmental Policy at

San Diego State University. He also holds an MA in Leadership Studies from the University of San Diego. He is the author of *The Adventures of Enu* and *Ashes in the Ocean*.

An East Coast native, Sonya grew up exploring the forests and fields in a suburb outside of Philadelphia, Pennsylvania. From an early age she pursued her passion for soccer, which eventually led her to play for the Seahawks at the University of North Carolina at Wilmington. After finishing her undergraduate studies, she enjoyed living and working across the U.S. and abroad. Sonya worked in higher education for over fifteen years at the University of North Carolina–Wilmington, Duke University, the University of California–Los Angeles (UCLA), and the University of San Diego (USD). She received her MEd in Student Affairs from UCLA and her MA in Leadership Studies from USD.

The married couple live and work together in the coastal town of Encinitas, California. When they are not writing or working on Nature Unplugged, the two enjoy exploring the many natural wonders around their home along with regular (and often intense) bouts of ping-pong.

FOR MORE INFORMATION

Visit www.natureunplugged.com and join the movement.

- Learn more about our work and services.
- Access podcasts and videos for more tips, tools, and takeaways.
- Download free worksheets and resources.
- See our schedule of speaking events and workshops.
- Join us for a retreat or excursion.
- Visit our store for books, products, and courses.

To connect with the authors directly, email:
sebastian@natureunplugged.com | sonya@natureunplugged.com

NOTES

INTRODUCTION: EXPERIENCE NATURE UNPLUGGED

1   Victoria Rideout and Michael B. Robb, *The Common Sense Census: Media Use by Tweens and Teens, 2019* (San Francisco, CA: Common Sense Media, 2019), https://www.commonsensemedia. org/sites/default/files/uploads/research/2019-census-8-to-18-key-findings-updated.pdf.

2   Neil E. Klepeis et al., "The National Human Activity Pattern Survey (NHAPS): A Resource for Assessing Exposure to Environmental Pollutants," Lawrence Berkeley National Laboratory and Environmental Health Sciences, School of Public Health, University of California at Berkeley (2001): 17, https://indoor.lbl.gov/ sites/all/files/lbnl-47713.pdf.

3   Common Sense Media, "New Report Finds Teens Feel Addicted to Their Phones, Causing Tension at Home," news release, May 3, 2016, https://www.commonsensemedia.org/about-us/news/ press-releases/new-report-finds-teens-feel-addicted-to-their-phones-causing-tension-at.

4   IDC Research Report, "Always Connected: How Smartphones and Social Keep Us Engaged," 2013, https://www.nu.nl/files/ IDC-Facebook%20Always%20Connected%20(1).pdf.

5   Craig M. Hales, Margaret D. Carroll, Cheryl D. Fryar, and Cynthia L. Ogden, "Prevalence of Obesity Among Adults and Youth: United States, 2015–2016," CDC/NCHS Data Brief No. 288, October 2017, https://www.cdc.gov/nchs/data/databriefs/db288. pdf.

6   Jean M. Twenge, Thomas E. Joiner, Megan L. Rogers, and Gabrielle N. Martin, "Increases in Depressive Symptoms, Suicide-Related Outcomes, and Suicide Rates Among U.S. Adolescents After 2010 and Links to Increased New Media Screen Time," *Clinical Psychological Science* 6, no. 1 (January 2018): 3–17, https://doi. org/10.1177/2167702617723376.

7   Jacqueline A. Sparks and Barry L. Duncan, "The Ethics and Science of Medicating Children," *Ethical Human Psychology and*

Psychiatry 6, no. 1 (Spring 2004): 25–39, http://www.psych-rights.org/research/Digest/ADHD/MedicatingKids.pdf.

8   *The Adventures of Enu: The Tale of the Giant Whale* (Nature Unplugged, 2012).

9   *Ashes in the Ocean: A Son's Story of Living Through and Learning from His Father's Suicide* (Nature Unplugged, 2018).

CHAPTER 1: CHALLENGES OF LIVING IN THE DIGITAL AGE

10   Rideout and Robb, *Common Sense Census.*

11   Rideout and Robb, *Common Sense Census.*

12   Child Mind Institute, *Talking to Tweens and Teens about Their Online Lives: A Supplement to the Children's Mental Health Report*, 2019, https://childmind.org/our-impact/childrens-mental-health-report/2019report/. Download the Parent Supplement.

13   Pew Research Center, "Mobile Fact Sheet," June 12, 2019, https://www.pewresearch.org/internet/fact-sheet/mobile/.

14   Andrew Perrin and Madhu Kumar, "About three-in-ten U.S. adults say they are 'almost constantly' online," Pew Research Center, July 25, 2019, https://www.pewresearch.org/fact-tank/2019/07/25/americans-going-online-almost-constantly/.

15   Perrin and Kumar, "About three-in-ten U.S. adults."

16   Jean M. Twenge, "Have Smartphones Destroyed a Generation?" *The Atlantic*, September 2017 Issue, https://www.theatlantic.com/magazine/archive/2017/09/has-the-smartphone-destroyed-a-generation/534198/.

17   Twenge, "Have Smartphones Destroyed a Generation?"

18   Child Mind Institute, *Talking to Tweens and Teens.*

19   Lars Louis Andersen and Anne Helene Garde, "Sleep problems and computer use during work and leisure: Cross-sectional study among 7800 adults," *Chronobiology International* 32, no. 10 (2015): 1367–1372, doi: 10.3109/07420528.2015.1095202

20   Geir Scott Brunborg et al., "The relationship between media use in the bedroom, sleep habits and symptoms of insomnia,"

Journal of Sleep Research 20 (2011): 569–575, https://doi. org/10.1111/j.1365-2869.2011.00913.x

21 Liese Exelmans and Jan Van den Bulck, "Bedtime mobile phone use and sleep in adults," *Social Science & Medicine* 148 (2016): 93–101, https://doi.org/10.1016/j.socscimed.2015.11.037.

22 Child Mind Institute, *Talking to Tweens and Teens.*

23 Child Mind Institute, *Talking to Tweens and Teens.*

24 Twenge, "Have Smartphones Destroyed a Generation?"

25 Brian A. Primack et al., "Social Media Use and Perceived Social Isolation Among Young Adults in the U.S.," *American Journal of Preventive Medicine* 53, no. 1 (July 2017): 1–8, https://doi. org/10.1016/j.amepre.2017.01.010.

26 "Nutrition, Physical Activity, and Obesity," healthypeople.gov (website), last modified October 8, 2020, https://www.healthypeople.gov/2020/leading-health-indicators/2020-lhi-topics/ Nutrition-Physical-Activity-and-Obesity#3.

27 "2020 Physical Activity Council's Overview Report on U.S. Participation," Physical Activity Council, 2020, https://eb6d91a4-d249-47b8-a5cb-933f7971db54.filesusr.com/ugd/286de6_c28995b76cf94de2a22ac7a0a4d5264d.pdf.

28 Craig M. Hales, Margaret D. Carroll, Cheryl D. Fryar, and Cynthia L. Ogden, "Prevalence of Obesity and Severe Obesity Among Adults: United States, 2017–2018," CDC/NCHS Data Brief No. 360, February 2020, https://www.cdc.gov/nchs/data/data-briefs/db360-h.pdf.

29 "Obesity and Overweight," CDC/National Center for Health Statistics, last reviewed February 28, 2020, https://www.cdc.gov/ nchs/fastats/obesity-overweight.htm.

30 Ewa Gustafsson, Sara Thomee, Anna Grimby-Ekman, and Mats Hagberg, "Texting on mobile phones and musculoskeletal disorders in young adults: A five-year cohort study," *Applied Ergonomics* 58 (January 2017): 208–214, https://doi.org/10.1016/j. apergo.2016.06.012.

31 Trevor Haynes, "Dopamine, Smartphones & You: A battle for

your time," Science in the News (blog), Harvard University, May 1, 2018, http://sitn.hms.harvard.edu/flash/2018/dopamine-smartphones-battle-time/.

32 J. Clement, "Number of active advertisers on Facebook from 1st quarter 2016 to 2nd quarter 2020," Statista (website), August 10, 2020, https://www.statista.com/statistics/778191/active-facebook-advertisers/#:~:text=Number%20of%20active%20advertisers%20on%20Facebook%202016%2D2020&text=In%20the%20second%20quarter%20of,quarter%20of%20the%20previous%20year.

33 Rishi Iyengar, "Here's how big Facebook's ad business really is," CNN Business, July 1, 2020, https://www.cnn.com/2020/06/30/tech/facebook-ad-business-boycott/index.html.

34 Chris Weller, "Silicon Valley parents are raising their kids tech-free—and it should be a red flag," *Business Insider*, February 18, 2018, https://www.businessinsider.com/silicon-valley-parents-raising-their-kids-tech-free-red-flag-2018-2.

35 Canela López, "6 tech executives who raise their kids tech-free or seriously limit their screen time," *Business Insider*, March 5, 2020, https://www.businessinsider.com/tech-execs-screen-time-children-bill-gates-steve-jobs-2019-9.

36 Matt Richtel, "A Silicon Valley School That Doesn't Compute," *New York Times*, October 22, 2011, https://www.nytimes.com/2011/10/23/technology/at-waldorf-school-in-silicon-valley-technology-can-wait.html.

CHAPTER 2: LEADERSHIP IN THE DIGITAL AGE

37 E. P. Hollander and J. W. Julian, "Contemporary trends in the analysis of leadership processes," *Psychological Bulletin* 71, no. 5 (1969): 387–397; K. K. Smith and D. N. Berg, *Paradoxes of Group Life* (San Francisco, CA: Jossey Bass, 1987); Ronald A. Heifetz, *Leadership Without Easy Answers* (Cambridge, MA: Harvard University Press, 1994).

38 Ronald A. Heifetz, Marty Linsky, and Alexander Grashow, *The*

Practice of Adaptive Leadership: Tools and Tactics for Changing Your Organization and the World (Boston, MA: Harvard Business Press, 2009), 22.

CHAPTER 3: WELLNESS WITH TECHNOLOGY

39 David Sax, "Our Love Affair With Digital Is Over," *New York Times*, November 18, 2017, https://www.nytimes.com/2017/11/18/opinion/sunday/internet-digital-technology-return-to-analog.html.

40 Pam A. Mueller and Daniel M. Oppenheimer, "The Pen Is Mightier Than the Keyboard: Advantages of Longhand Over Laptop Note Taking," *Psychological Science* 25, no. 6 (June 2014): 1159–1168. https://doi.org/10.1177/0956797614524581.

CHAPTER 4: A NATURAL SOLUTION

41 "2019 Outdoor Participation Report," Outdoor Foundation, January 29, 2020, https://outdoorindustry.org/resource/2019-outdoor-participation-report/.

42 Neil E. Klepeis et al., "The National Human Activity Pattern Survey (NHAPS): a resource for assessing exposure to environmental pollutants," *Journal of Exposure Science & Environmental Epidemiology* 11 (2001): 231–252, https://doi.org/10.1038/sj.jea.7500165.

43 Stephen Kaplan, "The Restorative Benefits of Nature: Toward an Integrative Framework," *Journal of Environmental Psychology* 15 (1995): 169–182, https://willsull.net/resources/KaplanS1995.pdf

44 Heather Ohly et al., "Attention Restoration Theory: A systematic review of the attention restoration potential of exposure to natural environments," *Journal of Toxicology and Environmental Health, Part B, Critical Reviews* 19, no. 7 (2016): 305–343, doi: 10.1080/10937404.2016.1196155.

45 Andrea Faber Taylor and Frances E. Kuo, "Children with attention deficits concentrate better after walk in the park," *Journal of Attention Disorders* 12, no. 5 (2009): 402–409, doi:

10.1177/1087054708323000.

46 Marc G. Berman, John Jonides, and Stephen Kaplan, "The Cognitive Benefits of Interacting With Nature," *Psychological Science* 19 (2008): 1207, doi: 10.1111/j.1467-9280.2008.02225.x.

47 Matthew Wichrowski, Jonathan Whiteson, François Haas, Ana Mola, and Mariano J. Rey, "Effects of horticultural therapy on mood and heart rate in patients participating in an inpatient cardiopulmonary rehabilitation program," *Journal of Cardiopulmonary Rehabilitation* 25, no. 5 (September–October 2005): 270–274, doi: 10.1097/00008483-200509000-00008.

48 "Nature Can Improve Health and Well-being," Children and Nature Network, 2016, https://www.childrenandnature.org/wp-content/uploads/CNN_NatureImprove_16-10-27_O_newlogo.pdf.

49 Huibrie C. Pieters, Leilanie Ayala, Ariel Schneider, Nancy Wicks, Aimee Levine-Dickman, and Susan Clinton, "Gardening on a psychiatric inpatient unit: Cultivating recovery," *Archives of Psychiatric Nursing* 33, no. 1 (February 2019): 57–64, https://doi.org/10.1016/j.apnu.2018.10.001.

50 Kirsten M. M. Beyer et al., "Exposure to neighborhood green space and mental health: evidence from the survey of the health of Wisconsin," *International Journal of Environmental Research and Public Health* 11, no. 3 (2014): 3453–3472, doi: 10.3390/ijerph110303453.

51 Ohly et al., "Attention Restoration Theory."

52 Q. Li et al., "Forest bathing enhances human natural killer activity and expression of anti-cancer proteins," *International Journal of Immunopathology and Pharmacology* 20, 2 Suppl. 2 (April–June 2007), 3–8. https://doi.org/10.1177/03946320070200S202.

53 Ruth Ann Atchley, David L. Strayer, and Paul Atchley, "Creativity in the Wild: Improving Creative Reasoning through Immersion in Natural Settings," *PLoS One* 7 (2012), https://doi.org/10.1371/journal.pone.0051474.

54 "Nature Can Improve Health and Well-being," Children and Nature Network.

55 Calum Neill, Janelle Gerard, and Katherine D. Arbuthnott, "Nature contact and mood benefits: contact duration and mood type," *The Journal of Positive Psychology* 14, no. 6 (2019): 756–767, https://doi.org/10.1080/17439760.2018.1557242.

56 Florence Williams, "Call to the Wild: This Is Your Brain on Nature," *National Geographic*, January 2016, https://www.nationalgeographic.com/magazine/2016/01/call-to-wild/ (paywall).

57 Gregory N. Bratman, J. Paul Hamilton, Kevin S. Hahn, Gretchen C. Daily, and James J. Gross, "Nature reduces rumination and sgPFC activation," *Proceedings of the National Academy of Sciences* (June 29, 2015), doi: 10.1073/pnas.1510459112.

58 Mathew P. White et al., "Spending at least 120 minutes a week in nature is associated with good health and wellbeing," *Scientific Reports* 9, no. 7730 (2019), https://doi.org/10.1038/s41598-019-44097-3.

59 Atchley, Strayer, and Atchley, "Creativity in the Wild."

CHAPTER 5: MOVEMENT

60 Obesity and Overweight Fact Sheet, World Health Organization, April 1, 2020, https://www.who.int/news-room/fact-sheets/detail/obesity-and-overweight.

61 Victoria J. Rideout, Ulla G. Foehr, and Donald F. Roberts, "Generation M2: Media in the Lives of 8- to 18-Year-Olds," Henry J. Kaiser Family Foundation, 2010, https://files.eric.ed.gov/fulltext/ED527859.pdf.

62 "Youth Risk Behavior Surveillance Summary, 2011," Centers for Disease Control and Prevention, https://www.cdc.gov/mmwr/preview/mmwrhtml/ss6104a1.htm.

63 "Physical Activity," U.S. Department of Health and Human Services (HHS), Office of Disease Prevention and Health Promotion, last modified October 8, 2020, https://www.healthypeople.gov/2020/topics-objectives/topic/physical-activity.

64 Y. Claire Wang, Klim McPherson, Tim Marsh, Steven L. Gort-maker, and Martin Brown, "Health and Economic Burden of the Projected Obesity Trends in the USA and the UK," *The Lancet* 378 (2011): 815–825, doi: 10.1016/S0140-6736(11)60814-3.

65 U.S. Department of Agriculture and U.S. Department of Health and Human Services, *Dietary Guidelines for Americans, 2010*, 7th ed. (Washington, DC: U.S. Government Printing Office, December 2010).

66 Gavin R. H. Sandercock and Daniel D. Cohen, "Temporal trends in muscular fitness of English 10-year-olds 1998–2014: An allometric approach," *Journal of Science and Medicine in Sport* 22, no. 2 (February 2019): 201–205, https://doi.org/10.1016/j. jsams.2018.07.020.

67 Arthur S. Leon et al., "Cardiac Rehabilitation and Second-ary Prevention of Coronary Heart Disease," *Circulation* 111, no. 3 (January 2005): 369–376, https://doi.org/10.1161/01. CIR.0000151788.08740.5C

68 J. A. Halbert et al., "The effectiveness of exercise training in low-ering blood pressure: a meta-analysis of randomised controlled trials of 4 weeks or longer," *Journal of Human Hypertension* 11 (1997): 641–649, doi: 10.1038/sj.jhh.1000509.

69 J. L. Durstine and W. L. Haskell, "Effects of exercise training on plasma lipids and lipoproteins," *Exercise and Sport Scienc-es Reviews* 22 (1994): 477–521, https://pubmed.ncbi.nlm.nih. gov/7925552/

70 Elizabeth Anderson and Geetha Shivakumar, "Effects of Exer-cise and Physical Activity on Anxiety," *Frontiers in Psychiatry* 4 (2013): 27, https://doi.org/10.3389/fpsyt.2013.00027

71 Johanna Takács, "Regular physical activity and mental health. The role of exercise in the prevention of, and intervention in depressive disorders," *Psychiatria Hungarica: A Magyar Pszichiatriai Tarsasag tudomanyos folyoirata* 29, no. 4 (2014): 386–397, https://pubmed.ncbi.nlm.nih.gov/25569828/

72 Gary M. Cooney et al., "Exercise for depression," *The Cochrane*

Database of Systematic Reviews 9 (2013), https://doi.org/10.1002/14651858.CD004366.pub6

73 Kathryn M. Fritz and Patrick J. O'Connor, "Acute Exercise Improves Mood and Motivation in Young Men with ADHD Symptoms," *Medicine and Science in Sports and Exercise* 48, no. 6 (2016): 1153–1160, https://doi.org/10.1249/ MSS.0000000000000864

74 Peter Payne and Mardi A. Crane-Godreau, "Meditative movement for depression and anxiety," *Frontiers in Psychiatry* 4, no. 71 (2013), https://doi.org/10.3389/fpsyt.2013.00071

75 Joanne Lumsden, Lynden K. Miles, and C. Neil Macrae, "Sync or sink? Interpersonal synchrony impacts self-esteem," *Frontiers in Psychology* 5, no. 1064 (2014), https://doi.org/10.3389/ fpsyg.2014.01064

76 "Walking for Health," Harvard Medical School Special Report, n.d., https://www.health.harvard.edu/exercise-and-fitness/walking-for-health.

77 "Exercise for Your Bone Health," National Institutes of Health: Osteoporosis and Related Bone Diseases, National Resource Center, October 2018, https://www.bones.nih.gov/sites/bones/files/ pdfs/exercisebonehealth-508.pdf.

78 A. D. Pellegrini and C. M. Bohn, "The role of recess in children's cognitive performance and school adjustment," *Educational Researcher* 34, no. 1 (2005): 13–19.

79 Jo Barton and Jules N. Pretty, "What is the Best Dose of Nature and Green Exercise for Improving Mental Health? A Multi-Study Analysis," *Environmental Science and Technology* 44, no. 10 (March 2010): 3947–3955, doi: 10.1021/es903183r

80 Gunnthora Olafsdottir et al., "Health Benefits of Walking in Nature: A Randomized Controlled Study Under Conditions of Real-Life Stress," *Environment and Behavior* (2018): 1–27, https:// doi.org/10.1177/0013916518800798.

81 Katharine Reed et al., "A repeated measures experiment of green exercise to improve self-esteem in UK school children," *PloS*

One 8, no. 7 (2013): e69176, https://doi.org/10.1371/journal. pone.0069176

82 Qing Li et al, "Acute effects of walking in forest environments on cardiovascular and metabolic parameters," *European Journal of Applied Physiology* (2011): 2845–2853, doi 10.1007/s00421-011-1918-z

83 Stella-Maria Hug, Terry Hartig, Ralf Hansmann, Klaus Seeland, and Rainer Hornung, "Restorative qualities of indoor and outdoor exercise settings as predictors of exercise frequency," *Health & Place* 15, no. 4 (2009), 971–980, https://doi.org/10.1016/j. healthplace.2009.03.002

84 Jo Barton and Jules Pretty, "What is the Best Dose of Nature and Green Exercise for Improving Mental Health? A Multi-Study Analysis," *Environmental Science & Technology* 44, no. 10 (March 2010): 3947–3955, doi: 10.1021/es903183r

CHAPTER 6: COMMUNITY AND CONNECTION

85 Johann Hari, *Chasing the Scream: The Opposite of Addiction Is Connection* (London: Bloomsbury, 2019).

86 Nicholas Epley and Juliana Schroeder, "Mistakenly Seeking Solitude," *Journal of Experimental Psychology: General* 143 no. 5 (2014): 1980–1999, https://doi.org/10.1037/a0037323

87 Henry Bawkin, "Emotional deprivation in infants," *The Journal of Pediatrics* 35, no. 4 (October 1949): 512–521, https://doi. org/10.1016/S0022-3476(49)80071-0.

88 Cal Newport, *Digital Minimalism: Choosing a Focused Life in a Noisy World* (London: Penguin Business, 2019).

89 Michael J. Mallen, Susan X. Day, and Melinda A. Green, "Online versus face-to-face conversation: An examination of relational and discourse variables," *Psychotherapy: Theory, Research, Practice, Training* 40, no. 1–2 (2003): 155–163, https://doi. org/10.1037/0033-3204.40.1-2.155

90 Sherry Turkle in Lauren Cassani Davis, "The Flight From Conversation," *The Atlantic*, October 7, 2015, https://www.theatlantic.

com/technology/archive/2015/10/reclaiming-conversation-sher-ry-turkle/409273/

CHAPTER 7: MINDFULNESS

91 Alvin Powell, "When Science Meets Mindfulness," *The Harvard Gazette*, April 9, 2018, https://news.harvard.edu/gazette/story/2018/04/harvard-researchers-study-how-mindfulness-may-change-the-brain-in-depressed-patients/.

92 Manoj K. Bhasin et al., "Specific Transcriptome Changes Associated with Blood Pressure Reduction in Hypertensive Patients After Relaxation Response Training," *Journal of Alternative and Complementary Medicine* 24, no. 5 (2018); 486–504, https://doi.org/10.1089/acm.2017.0053

93 Mike Vorkunov, "Coached by the Zen Master, the Knicks Try Mindfulness," *New York Times*, December 6, 2016, https://www.nytimes.com/2016/12/06/sports/basketball/phil-jackson-zen-master-knicks-mindfulness.html.

94 Hugh Delehanty, "The Game Changer: How Seattle Seahawks Coach Pete Carroll is Reshaping NFL Culture," *Mindful*, December 22, 2014, https://www.mindful.org/the-game-changer/.

95 *The Adventures of Enu: The Tale of the Giant Whale* (Nature Unplugged, 2012).

CHAPTER 8: MINDSET

96 Carol S. Dweck, *Mindset: The New Psychology of Success*, updated ed. (New York: Ballantine, 2016).

CHAPTER 9: INNER ALIGNMENT

97 Tim Kasser and Richard M. Ryan, "Be careful what you wish for: Optimal functioning and the relative attainment of intrinsic and extrinsic goals," in Peter Schmuck and Kennon M. Sheldon, eds., *Life Goals and Well-Being: Towards a Positive Psychology of Human Striving* (Seattle, WA: Hogrefe & Huber, 2001), 116–131.

98 Sonja Lyubomirsky, *The How of Happiness: A New Approach to*

Getting the Life You Want (New York: Penguin, 2008).

99   Johann Hari, *Lost Connections: Uncovering the Real Causes of Depression—and the Unexpected Solutions* (Bloomsbury USA, 2018).

100 Johann Hari, "We know junk food makes us sick. Are 'junk values' making us depressed?" *Los Angeles Times*, op-ed, January 21, 2018, https://www.latimes.com/opinion/op-ed/la-oe-hari-kasser-junk-values-20180121-story.html.

101 Tim Kasser, Richard M. Ryan, Charles E. Couchman, and Kennon M. Sheldon, "Materialistic values: Their causes and consequences," in T. Kasser and A. D. Kanner, eds., *Psychology and Consumer Culture: The Struggle for a Good Life in a Materialistic World* (American Psychological Association, 2004), 11–28, https://doi.org/10.1037/10658-002.

102 *Oxford Dictionary* (Lexico), s.v. "FOMO," accessed November 29, 2020, https://www.lexico.com/en/definition/fomo.

CHAPTER 10: PLAY

103 Martin Seligman and Mihaly Csikszentmihalyi, "Positive psychology: An introduction," *American Psychologist* 55, no. 1 (2000): 5–14, https://doi.org/10.1037/0003-066X.55.1.5.

104 Jeffrey J. Froh, "The History of Positive Psychology: Truth Be Told," *The Psychologist* 16, no. 3 (May/June 2004): 18–20, https://scottbarrykaufman.com/wp-content/uploads/2015/01/Froh-2004.pdf.

105 Christopher Peterson, "What is positive psychology, and what is it not?" *Psychology Today* (2008) in Courtney E. Ackerman, "What is Positive Psychology & Why is It Important?" PositivePsychology.com, October 19, 2020, https://positivepsychology.com/what-is-positive-psychology-definition/.

106 Research compiled in "Play Facts," The Genius of Play (website), n.d., https://thegeniusofplay.org/tgop/benefits/play-facts/genius/benefits-of-play/facts/play-facts.aspx.

107 "Play Facts," The Genius of Play (website).

108 "Play Facts," The Genius of Play (website).

109 "Play Facts," The Genius of Play (website).

110 Stuart L. Brown and Christopher C. Vaughan, *Play: How It Shapes the Brain, Opens the Imagination, and Invigorates the Soul* (New York: Avery, 2009).

111 "Loss of Open Space," U.S. Forest Service (website), n.d., https://www.fs.usda.gov/science-technology/loss-of-open-space.

112 Pew Research Center, "U.S. violent and property crime rate have plunged since 1990s, regardless of data source," November 20, 2020, https://www.pewresearch.org/fact-tank/2020/11/20/facts-about-crime-in-the-u-s/ft_20-11-12_crimeintheus_2/

113 Amanda Rock, "Unstructured Play for Children," verywellfamily.com, September 17, 2020, https://www.verywellfamily.com/unstructured-play-2764971.

114 Alison Gopnik, "In Defense of Play," *The Atlantic*, August 12, 2016, https://www.theatlantic.com/education/archive/2016/08/in-defense-of-play/495545/.

CHAPTER 11: CREATIVITY

115 Christopher G. Lucas, Sophie Bridgers, Thomas L. Griffiths, and Alison Gopnik, "When children are better (or at least more open-minded) learners than adults: developmental differences in learning the forms of causal relationships," *Cognition* 131, no. 2 (2014): 284–299, https://doi.org/10.1016/j.cognition.2013.12.010.

116 Grant Hilary Brenner, "Your Brain on Creativity," *Psychology Today*, February 22, 2018, https://www.psychologytoday.com/us/blog/experimentations/201802/your-brain-creativity

117 Girija Kaimal, Kendra Ray, and Juan Muniz, "Reduction of Cortisol Levels and Participants' Responses Following Art Making," *Art Therapy* 33, no. 2 (2016): 74–80, doi: 10.1080/07421656.2016.1166832

118 Heather L. Stuckey and Jeremy Nobel, "The connection between art, healing, and public health: a review of current literature," *American Journal of Public Health* 100, no. 2 (2010): 254–263, https://doi.org/10.2105/AJPH.2008.156497

119 Stuckey and Nobel, "The connection between art, healing, and public health."

120 Jennifer E. Graham, Marci Lobel, Peter Glass, and Irina Lokshina, "Effects of written anger expression in chronic pain patients: making meaning from pain," *Journal of Behavioral Medicine* 31 (2008): 201–212, https://doi.org/10.1007/s10865-008-9149-4

121 American Friends of Tel Aviv University, "Teaching creativity to children from a galaxy away," EurekAlert! (American Association for the Advancement of Science news release), May 17, 2012, https://www.eurekalert.org/pub_releases/2012-05/afot-tct051712.php

122 Aimee Groth, "The Moment When Marc Benioff Came Up With The Idea For Salesforce.com," *Business Insider*, October 21, 2011, https://www.businessinsider.com/marc-benioff-salesforcecom-innovators-dna-2011-10.

CONCLUSION: ENGAGED LIVING

123 *Living with the Amish* (UK: KEO Films, 2011), six-part documentary series.

124 Jeff Brady, "Amish Community Not Anti-Technology, Just More Thoughtful," NPR, September 2, 2013, https://www.npr.org/sections/alltechconsidered/2013/09/02/217287028/amish-community-not-anti-technology-just-more-thoughful.